# LIGHT HER FIRE

ALSO BY ELLEN KREIDMAN

*LIGHT HIS FIRE:*
*How to Keep Your Man*
*Passionately and Hopelessly*
*in Love with You*

# LIGHT HER FIRE

*How to Ignite Passion and Excitement in the Woman You Love*

ELLEN KREIDMAN

*Villard Books*
*1991*

 Published in the United States by Villard Books, a division of Random House, Inc., New York, and simultaneously in Canada by Random House of Canada Limited, Toronto.



Library of Congress Cataloging-in-Publication Data
Kriedman, Ellen.
Light her fire:
how to ignite passion and
excitement in the woman
you love/by Ellen Kriedman.
p. cm.
ISBN 0-394-58802-9
1. Sex instruction for men. 2. Love. 3. Women—Psychology.
I. Title.
HQ36.K74 1990
613.9'6—dc20 90-50219

Manufactured in the United States of America
9 8 7 6 5 4 3 2
First Edition

# DEDICATION

This book is dedicated to my husband, Steve, who lit my fire the first day I met him in high school more than thirty years ago and has kept the flame of passion burning throughout our twenty-four years of marriage.

# WARNING!!!

**Do not read this book unless you are a man who wants:**

- Nights of sensuous pleasure
- Adventure beyond your wildest fantasies
- To experience the delight in unleashing unpredictable, spontaneous behavior
- An exciting, passionate lover
- True intimacy
- A compassionate, understanding, and responsive woman
- To become the man most women only dream about

I REPEAT, do not under any circumstances, read this book unless you sincerely want to ignite the flame of passion in the woman you love!

# A NOTE FROM THE AUTHOR

## CONSIDER IT A COMPLIMENT

There are several ways this book may have come into your possession:

You bought *Light Her Fire* yourself, and in that case, congratulations. You are a very special man and deserve to be commended for your desire to become the best possible lover and mate.

A friend gave you *Light Her Fire,* a friend who has found something very special and can't help sharing it with people he or she cares about.

*Light Her Fire* was a present from your girlfriend or wife. Consider it the ultimate compliment. What she's saying is, "You are the most important person in my life, and I love you deeply. I want us to have all the happiness that we deserve. I don't want to settle for a mediocre, run-of-the-mill, average relationship. I want us to join the ranks of great lovers. I know I seem unlovable and impossible at times, but if you'll take the time to understand what my needs are, I'll do the same for you. Then we can have a relationship filled with passion, excitement, and sexual fulfillment."

Your mother may have given you *Light Her Fire* because she desperately wants you to be happy. No matter how old you are, you will always be her child, and her natural instinct is to want to protect you against disappointment and pain. Be grateful that you have someone who wants you to have only the best that life has to offer.

I promise that if you will take a few hours to read this material, you will have all the knowledge necessary to become your woman's knight in shining armor. You will be her hero forever, and you will have at your fingertips everything you need to say and do to have her respond to you in a way you never dreamed possible.

- If you are single, you will have more women in your life than you know what to do with. They will find you irresistible. You will be leaps and bounds ahead of any competition you might have had before.
- If you've been hurt in a past relationship and are nervous about entering a new one, rest assured that you will have the confidence it takes to begin again. And, what's even more important, you will understand what went wrong and won't be so prone to make the same mistakes you made before.
- If you have a girlfriend, she'll want you to be her partner for the rest of your lives. You'll remove all doubts she may have had.
- If you are married to an unresponsive woman, look out! She will respond!

- If you are getting divorced, you will be surprised at how easy it is to repair a damaged relationship.
- If you are happily married, you'll know how to keep forever what you have now.

Let's get started on this journey together, and learn how you can become everything that special woman ever dreamed of having in a man. In return, your fantasies will become a reality. Learn to ignite the flame of passion in her so that you can have an exciting, sensual, caring woman for the rest of your life.

Ellen Kreidman
January 1991

# ACKNOWLEDGMENTS

I am deeply grateful to the following people in my life who have given so much of themselves:

To my parents, who lit each other's fires for forty-seven and a half years and gave me a wonderful, secure childhood with many precious memories.

To my children, Tara, Tiffany, and Jason, who have created harmony and balance in my life.

To my brother and sister-in-law, Harvey and Susan, who have had a love affair with each other for sixteen years and have made me a proud aunt of their beautiful children, Matthew and Allison.

To my sister-in-law and brother-in-law, Barbara and Dale, who are living examples of the principles I teach.

To Frankie Wright, whose daily encouragement and enthusiasm helped expand my program. She has touched many lives with her honesty and compassion.

To Diane Reverend, my editor, whose wisdom, experience, guidance, and patience are a constant source of inspiration.

To Janet Bolen, my publicist, who has been a support system for the past two years. Her dedication, friendship, and ability to give of herself both personally and professionally motivated me to do and give the best I had to offer.

To Stevie Rimer, my office manager, whose ability to handle the daily activities with competence and enthusiasm has given me the freedom to concentrate on getting my message to a larger audience.

To the Irvine Hilton and Towers Hotel, which provided me with the service and tranquility necessary for creative thoughts to flow.

And most of all, to the men of my "Light Her Fire" seminars for taking time out to learn with me and to share their experiences. Without them, this book could not have been written.

# CONTENTS

# INTRODUCTION

## WHAT ABOUT US?

I had been teaching my "Light His Fire" course for women for several years before I finally decided to organize a class for men. My initial reason for the men's class was to satisfy all those women who asked, "Don't you have a course for men?" or "How do you expect me to take this class when there's nothing for him?"

I kept postponing the starting date because somewhere along the way I had accepted the common belief that men were not really interested in improving their relationships, that there was no way I was going to get a group of men to sit in a class one evening a week for five weeks in order to learn how to treat their women. I thought about a one-day seminar, then about a full five-week course, but that was about as far as it got. It was much easier to push the thoughts aside and postpone the whole idea than to begin something about which I had such doubts.

One day, I received a phone call from a man who was distraught because his wife wanted a divorce. She had fallen in love with a doctor she worked with at the hospital. I don't think I'll ever forget his voice when, after explaining the whole situation, he asked me, "What about us? Why don't you have a class that men can take? Don't we count too?" I could feel the pain in his voice and gave him what comfort I could. Again, I thought vaguely that I should soon offer that men's class.

Approximately two weeks later, I received another phone call, a desperate cry for help from a man who had just returned home from work to a vacant house. His wife had left him a note explaining that she and the children had gone to live with her mother in another state. She had had the movers come and take all their belongings, and was putting them in storage until she got herself settled. He had heard about my classes and some of the incredible results and wondered if he could sit in on the women's class, since there was nothing for men. "I'll do anything at this point to get her back," he cried.

A voice inside me said, "Ellen, what are you waiting for? Just do it!" I heard myself telling him, "That won't be necessary. The first men's class will begin in three weeks."

I sent out letters to all my female graduates announcing the first men's class and offering a reduction in price for their boyfriends, husbands, friends, or sons. I decided to hold the class for five weeks, on Saturday mornings from ten o'clock to noon.

## NO SIGN OF LIFE

On May 13, 1982, one year after the course for women, the first men's class was ready to begin. As they came in, I sensed an uncomfortable feeling permeating the room. I tried to make small talk while we waited for everyone to arrive, but none of them was receptive, thirty-five men, all cool and aloof, all wishing they were somewhere else.

As I introduced myself to the group and shared a little of my background, I was keenly aware that no one was looking at me. They were staring at their notebooks, pens, hands, out the window, anywhere but at me. I asked each man to introduce himself and tell the class why he was there. Of the thirty-five men, five were there because they had heard about the class and decided it was something from which they would benefit. The other thirty had joined because of ultimatums, threats, persuasion, or nagging. So the truth was that most of them did not want to be there. They had shown up just to please their wives or girlfriends, to get them off their backs.

Halfway through the lesson, I realized I was as uncomfortable teaching as they were being there. When we took a fifteen-minute break, every man, without exception, left the room to get some fresh air. They scurried out of that room as fast as they could, leaving me alone to gaze out the window at them. Some of them began smoking and staring out into the parking lot. Others were pacing back and forth, and still others were staring down at the sidewalk. Not one man spoke to another. There was complete silence. It seemed as if each of those men had his space, and you didn't dare invade his privacy. That was exactly what I had been doing for the past hour.

Somehow I got through the rest of the class. When it was over, there was a mad dash for the front door, no good-byes or acknowledgments, just an empty feeling in the pit of my stomach that I had done a terrible job. What a difference there was between the men's and women's classes. The women's classes always began with a great deal of noise as the women eagerly introduced themselves to me and their classmates. I always had to bang the microphone several times to signal that conversation had to stop, that I was ready to begin. At the breaks, several women always came up immediately, asking me questions or commenting on what I had said. Laughter, anticipation, and camaraderie were evident throughout the entire class. When the lesson was over, I'd end up staying at least an hour more, since some of the women always had questions, comments, and stories to supplement the class.

The next Saturday, I left home feeling as if I wanted to be anywhere but in that classroom. To my amazement, several men had arrived early to chat. They had been thinking all week about what they learned and had some thoughts to share. Others brought in magazine articles that supported what I had discussed and which they thought I might enjoy. A few even began talking to the men seated next to them. Lo and behold, there was life after all!

From then on, it was full steam ahead. The same laughter, participation, and camaraderie in the women's class was now evident in the men's class. It just took longer for the men to feel comfortable. They had been nervous and suspicious, not knowing what to expect, but they had learned that there was nothing threatening about my class and no reason to be defensive. They had nothing to defend, since I was not on the attack. I wasn't telling them they had been wrong all their lives: I was merely giving them a basis for better understanding. This was simply a class about understanding the woman with whom they would be spending the rest of their lives.

I think I learned as much from that first class as the men did. I learned that men are more guarded than women. It takes more time for them to feel comfortable with strangers. They are more cautious and not nearly as trusting, especially when it comes to discussing their private lives with strangers. And the best part of all was that I learned I was not a terrible teacher!

Since that first men's class nine years ago, I have taught thousands of men and have found each class to be a wonderful challenge. They've kept me on my toes. I've been able to fine-tune my style of teaching so that I'm more direct and get to the point faster. Men are not as accepting as women when generalizations are made; they want specific examples. The men in my classes have argued about and questioned, as well as supported and added to, my initial material. I was forced to grow in my ability as an instructor. I had to learn to present my information more clearly and concisely, and still be entertaining. I am forever grateful to all those men who have contributed to that process.

## THE CHALLENGE

As I traveled throughout the United States promoting my first book, *Light His Fire: How to Keep Your Man Passionately and Hopelessly in Love with You,* the overwhelming response from men from all walks of life was extremely positive. Many, for the first time in their lives, took the time to write (or call in, if I was appearing on a radio station) to say that they supported what I had to say one hundred percent. Never once in that one-year period, or in all the years that I have been teaching my classes, have I ever had a negative response from a man. Their reactions have always been the same.

> "How can I get my girlfriend or wife to read this?"
>
> "I can't believe my ears. Finally, someone is giving an accurate picture of what I have been missing most of my life."
>
> "After listening to you, I realize why I cheated on my wife and why I'm divorced now."

But not everyone was quite so bleak. Other men took the time to say they had been married for many years to a wonderful woman who does make them feel terrific, that they were living examples of a loving relationship. They confirmed that their wives had been doing what I taught.

*Light His Fire* became an instant national best-seller, yet I know there were many women who were reluctant to try it, thinking it was just "another book for women." Their response was, "Don't you have a book like this for men? Why does it always have to be the woman who finds out how to make a relationship work?"

In a society where one out of every two marriages ends in divorce, a man must be just as interested and committed to making his relationship work as is the woman in his life. I believe that a man cares every bit as much about fulfilling a woman's needs as she does about fulfilling his. What man would not want to have the "inside scoop" about what makes the other half of his relationship tick? A man, too, wants to know how to keep his mate hopelessly and passionately in love with him.

Up to now, there has been very little information written exclusively for you. I'm thrilled that I can offer you *Light Her Fire* as the companion book to hers. This book is for you, the man in your woman's life.

Please don't leave your personal life to luck or chance. You wouldn't do that with your career. If someone gave you an easy step-by-step program showing you exactly how to achieve success and wealth in your professional life, would you follow it? Of course you would. I'm giving you the same chance in your personal life. Based on my nine years of teaching men and women of all ages and varied backgrounds, together with a twenty-four-year love affair with the same man and experiencing three wonderful children who have grown to adulthood, I will give you everything you need to know to love a woman the way she deserves to be loved.

With some time, effort, and thought on your part, the rewards that await you are abundant.

Here are just a few examples of what has happened to some of the male graduates of my "Light Her Fire" seminars.

John reports, "My increased income has been a direct result of my newfound happiness with my wife. On the verge of my second divorce, I was making only a few hundred dollars a month. After 'Light Her Fire,' my wife and I became best friends as well as lovers. I felt so great about myself that my income went to a few thousand dollars a month!"

Your professional life is directly related to your personal

life. The happier you are at home, the more energy you have to devote to your job. A bad relationship is exhausting and drains you of the power you need to be successful. There is also much more reason to earn an exceptional income when you have an exceptional woman in your life!

Bob declares, "It's amazing how it takes eight hours a day to make my job a success, and all it took was a few minutes a day to turn my personal life around. I was ready to call it quits. As far as I was concerned, I had been cheated. The passionate women were only on the screen at the movies. My life at home was a living nightmare. My wife was wrapped up in her needs, her career, and gave absolutely nothing to me. I felt empty and alone for the past three years. Now I'm living what I thought was only possible in my fantasies. I can't wait to come home to the most romantic woman alive!"

Jim thinks there are no accidents in life. He had heard about "Light Her Fire" for two years from different sources before he finally decided that he'd take the gamble with his time and money and enroll. "I remember sitting in that class of thirty-five men and being the only one who was not in a serious relationship. I am twenty-six years old and up to now never had the feeling that I wanted to spend the rest of my life with any woman. My observations of my parents staying together in a loveless marriage, filled with anger and accusations, made me what I thought was a confirmed bachelor. I never knew that a union between two people could bring happiness. When I learned how easy it was to have a life with a woman who was caring and supportive, my anger and resentment of women disappeared. With my newfound understanding, I had the space to allow someone to come into my life. I'm now engaged to be married to the most fantastic woman. Now I know ways to avoid the pitfalls that my parents never knew."

Dan is another shining example of what understanding and insight into relationships can do for you. "I always felt unworthy of someone treating me with kindness and respect. I had developed a pattern. The three women in my life had all treated me badly, and I took it. It was as if I was saying, 'I'm worthless; therefore, I deserve what I get.' It was a self-fulfilling prophecy. When I learned what is possible in a healthy relationship with a woman, I was able to let go of someone in my life who was not worthy of my love. I now feel free and eager to find someone I can love and who loves me the way I deserve to be loved."

Last is Al, a newlywed. Every week he came in beaming. He was there at the request of his new bride, who had taken "Light His Fire." I had the sense that all the other men envied the excitement he felt in his new life. Nothing in Al's relationship was wrong. Each week he would give examples of what he or his wife was doing to support whatever I said. He was a reminder to all the other men in that class of what they may have had in the beginning but had lost somewhere along the way. He shared what he had learned, saying, "I will never take for granted that what we have today will be forever. My relationship will take work on a daily basis. I have the knowledge of how to keep my wife happy, glowing, and responsive. I don't want to be responsible for turning her into a cold, hard, uncaring woman." He thanked all the other men for "baring their souls" and reminding him how easy it is to assume that she would always be there for him, no matter what, even though that assumption might be completely wrong.

The principles I teach will work for you, too. In the last

nine years I've received hundreds of letters from happy, satisfied women who have taken the time to write and tell me what miraculous changes they've seen in their men. I'll begin each chapter with one of these letters so that you, too, can see the joy and excitement that have been inspired by some of the exceptional men who have learned to Light Her Fire.

Dear Ellen,

I want you to know that because Kurt took your class, I now have in my possession the most treasured gift I've ever gotten from him. For our eighteenth anniversary, he made a poster entitled "Why I Love My Wife." He listed eighteen reasons why he loves me. I cried the entire morning after getting this gift of love that came straight from his heart. It has a permanent spot in our bedroom right next to a wife who feels like a new bride. Thanks for the magic you perform.

Love,
Ellie

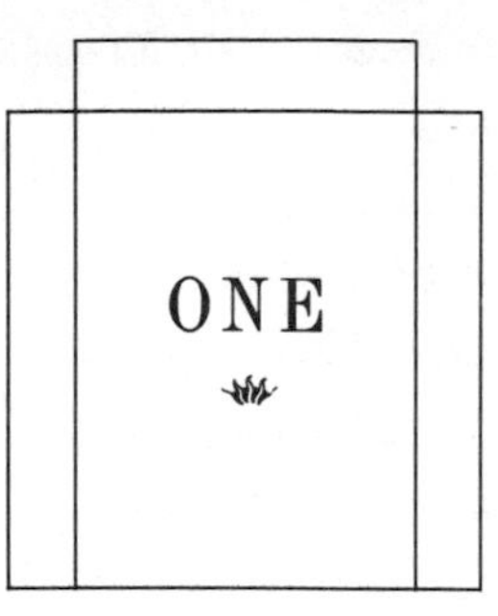

# A Toast to Your Differences

## AN EVENING TO REMEMBER

It began with a note, handwritten on exquisite gray linen stationery. Her heartbeat quickened at the faint scent of cologne coming from the envelope. She slowly opened the letter, savoring its beauty, and her surprise quickly turned into delight as she read. She was completely captivated by this note telling her she was the most desirable woman in the world. She read it over and over, not believing that she could ever have received something as romantic as this. After all, such things occurred only in her fantasies, in novels or movies. The note went on to tell her how valuable she was to his very existence, extolling her virtues, celebrating her uniqueness. She was wonderful, caring, beautiful, and smart, too. At the end was an invitation for a date on Friday evening at six-thirty. The address was very familiar. She had been living there for several years.

All week long, anticipation of her special evening occupied her mind. She passed the days smiling and humming without apparent reason.

When she arrived at the time and place specified in the

note, the lights were out, and candles were placed strategically throughout the house. A note pinned to the staircase read, "You've had an exhausting week, and you need to be pampered. Please come upstairs to the bathroom, where a soothing bath and an attendant await your pleasure." Her heart beat faster and faster as she climbed the stairs.

She opened the door to the bathroom and looked around in disbelief. A bubble bath was drawn, and rose petals were everywhere, floating in the water, carpeting the floor, permeating the room with soft fragrance. Beautiful flowerpots filled with azaleas, petunias, orchids, and daffodils had been placed here and there, and soft music played as though keeping time with the flicker of candlelight. He had transformed her rather ordinary bathroom into a haven of sensual tranquility.

Suddenly, she felt a gentle hand on her waist, and a voice whispered in her ear, "I want you to relax, unwind. Soak in the bath for a while. You deserve that. Then I'm going to give you a massage, head to toe."

She thought, "This is obviously a dream. It couldn't be happening. Any minute now, I'm going to wake up."

She undressed slowly and slipped into the tub, closing her eyes and languishing in the warmth, listening to the quiet music and allowing the soft fragrance of the flowers to fill her with flights of fancy.

As she finally arose from her bath, ready to step out onto the wonderful, soft carpet of rose petals, the door opened and the man she had known for thirty-two years stood before her in a kimono. He came to her and dried her gently with a warm towel, anointed her generously from a beautiful new bottle of perfume, then draped a kimono that matched his own about her shoulders.

He led her into the bedroom, which was bathed in candlelight and filled with vases of fresh-cut flowers, and asked her to dance. She melted into his arms and closed her eyes, wishing this moment would never end. They danced close and slow to the quiet music. How had he managed to find all her favorite songs?

After dancing for some time, he slowly, seductively led her to the bed, where he had chilled champagne waiting, along with a bottle of lotion. They toasted their luck, their life, their togetherness, their differences, and he took her glass and set it aside, then reached out a gentle hand and pulled the kimono from her shoulder. He smiled and rubbed the lotion in his hands to warm it before he stroked her slowly and gently from head to toe. This magnificent man whispered terms of endearment all the while, moving her, causing her heart to throb for him, the man of her dreams.

Sound like a scene in the movies or on a soap opera? It's not. This is just one of the romantic memories created from the "Light Her Fire" principles you are about to learn.

The players in the above story are John, fifty-seven, and Mary, fifty-three. They have been married for thirty-two years and have four grandchildren. John had never done anything like this, though he had always longed for something more from their relationship. For years, he had dreamed that Mary, a very shy, inhibited woman, would set the scene for their lovemaking.

When he took "Light Her Fire," he finally realized that he could be the one who took charge, that he could be the one who ignited the flame. He no longer had to wait for her to take the initiative. He learned that it was well within his power to teach her to let her imagination run wild. He could teach her to appreciate her own body, and he could teach her the fine art of seduction. These were all abilities he possessed and could carry out with the greatest of ease once he gave himself permission.

John told his entire class one evening, "I've never been a very good planner, and I was nervous about how she would react, but my wife's response was worth every bit of the time and effort I put into that evening. What a wonderful feeling it is to stop wishing and hoping for a woman to be someone she isn't and just love her for all the strengths she does have. I only wish I had done it thirty years ago."

## A TRUE PARTNERSHIP

A fulfilling partnership with a woman is only possible when both of you realize that the other person may think and do things differently, but that each of you has equal value and that each of you must respect the other's uniqueness. Whenever you attempt to create a carbon copy of yourself from another person, you lose. You lose the value and knowledge that your mate can contribute to your personal growth. The woman in your life has many lessons to teach you, just as you have many to teach her.

Remember, *if two people agree about everything, one of them is not necessary in the relationship.*

I have been an extrovert for as long as I can remember. I get energized when people are around me. When we first met, my husband was more introverted and enjoyed activities that required only the two of us. As a result, being with him all these years has taught me to be happy with or without people. I've learned to enjoy spending time by myself and not to rely so much on others' opinions. On the other hand, I have taught my husband how to be more social, and I've shown him the advantages of getting feedback from other people.

## THE NEVER-ENDING JOURNEY

When I first started my classes, I was always surprised when men or women in their seventies enrolled. The first day, I'd always have all the participants introduce themselves and explain in just a few sentences why they decided to take the class. Many of the senior citizens cited the following:

> "I figure you're never too old to learn something new."
>
> "If you don't keep growing, you die, and I'm not ready to call it quits just yet."
>
> "Honey, I may look old on the outside, but inside, there's still a young man who wants a woman to be attracted to him."
>
> "Every time when I think I know it all, along comes some tidbit of information that shocks the heck out of me and shows me that there's always something more I can learn."

I will never forget George. Here was a man seventy-eight years young telling me, "Sweetie, I live in Leisure World, where the women outnumber the men ten to one. There's so many women and so little time left. I want them all."

My response was, "You frisky little devil, good for you!"

All of these men were still eager to go on the never-ending journey of enlightenment. Personal growth is a life-long process. Even men in their seventies were attracted to my class because they somehow knew that a man who has a woman at his side receives more clarity, depth of understanding, and fulfillment in his life than if he lives alone. That's probably why statistics show that married men live much longer than single men.

## DIFFERENCES CAUSE GROWTH

It is not by chance, but by design, that opposites attract. Many men have contributed stories of the growth that came to them because of the wonderful women in their lives.

Paul didn't think he would ever have become as successful as he is today if it hadn't been for his wife, Marsha. "I was the logical, practical, analytical type. Marsha was a dreamer. I would probably still be working for someone else had she not convinced me that my abilities and talents were worth more than I thought and that I could afford to take risks. Her belief in me is what changed my attitude. Today, I am a real estate broker with four offices and ninety salespeople. We took out all the equity in our home, and I opened my first office ten years ago. I know if I had been by myself, I never would have done that. I started out as a messenger. I've changed a lot with her support."

Ted said he was a much more caring person because of the new girlfriend in his life. He saw changes taking place in just a few months of knowing Alice. Alice was a volunteer at a local hospital and convalescent home. Ted admitted, "When I first met Alice, I couldn't believe that anyone would do so much for free. I thought she had to be nuts! Then she invited me to go along with her one Saturday. Now, I'm hooked too! The people I met were so interesting and yet so lonely. I walked away realizing I received much more than I gave that day."

Kirk said, "I would have missed out on fatherhood completely if I hadn't met Betty. She had been widowed at a very young age and had two boys, aged one and three. You might say I got a package deal. I had never wanted children, because my childhood had been awful. I thought there were no paternal feelings in me at all. That's all changed now. I think I'm a good father to my boys. I've legally adopted them and can't imagine life without my family. Betty brought out feelings I never thought I'd be capable of experiencing."

I believe that opposites always attract: she makes you feel whole, and you do the same for her. She is your complement. People are like clay. There are only a few years in which you can mold the clay, probably only the first three or four. Then the clay hardens and holds its shape. You can try changing its beauty by taking a hammer and chisel to it, but all you'll really do is cause an ugly crack or break it. In the same way, you were attracted to your girlfriend or wife because of her uniqueness. You were excited by the very fact that she was different from you. Your sense of wonderment made her feel terrific. So why try to change her?

If you can appreciate her for who she is and find value in her uniqueness, she'll want to become more of a woman for you. There's nothing a woman won't do for a man who makes her feel good about herself.

## ACCENTUATE THE POSITIVE

Up to now, you may have been looking at some of her personality traits as bad, negative, or wrong. See if you can change your way of thinking by saying, "How would someone who really loves this woman view the same traits that have begun to annoy me?"

I'll help you with some suggestions, then you're on your own to add to the list.

Negative — She talks too much.
*Positive* — She's so friendly and puts everyone at ease.

Negative — She argues so much.
*Positive* — She has such strong convictions.

Negative — She thinks she knows it all.
*Positive* — She really is quite intelligent.

Negative — She's so conceited.
*Positive* — She has so much confidence in herself.

Negative — She's too easygoing.
*Positive* — She really has a calming effect on everyone.

Negative — She's so stingy.
*Positive* — She's trying to save money for our future.

Negative — She spends too much money.
*Positive* — She's always trying to improve our lifestyle.

Negative — She's too rigid.
*Positive* — She's really very organized.

Negative — She can never sit still.
*Positive* — She has so much energy.

Negative — She's too emotional.
*Positive* — She's so sensitive.

Clearly, it's not a woman's traits but how you view those traits that will determine how you react to them.

## TURN YOUR DIFFERENCES INTO COMPLIMENTS

A woman has to feel loved, needed, and accepted for who she is, and she has to feel appreciated for what she does. Give her these gifts in abundance, and you will get back her love, respect, admiration, and devotion. These gifts have to be given almost daily for her to get the assurance she needs. How do you give them? *You say them.* Your cost—nothing. Your reward—a woman who responds to your needs in return.

The following are areas of potential conflict viewed in a positive way.

If she enjoys people, and you don't, thank her for helping you not to be so judgmental toward everyone.

If she's practical, and you're a dreamer, tell her how wonderful it is to have a woman who keeps you grounded.

If she loves experiencing things, and you are result oriented, thank her for helping you enjoy the process, not necessarily the end product.

If she's bubbly and vivacious, and you are "doom and gloom," thank her for making you a more positive person.

If she's verbal, and you're a good listener, tell her how wonderful it is to have someone so entertaining and outgoing.

If she's spontaneous, and you are cautious, thank her for teaching you how to be less methodical and to enjoy the moment.

If she's adventuresome, and you are practical, thank her for making you less fearful and cautious.

If she's optimistic, and you are pessimistic, thank her for giving you hope and anticipation about the future.

If she's got charisma, and you are conservative, thank her for giving you inspiration and providing you with a woman who's exciting.

If she's responsible, and you are carefree, thank her for helping you become more organized and effective.

If she's imaginative, and you're more down-to-earth, thank her for helping you become more creative and playful.

If she's thorough and a stickler for details, and you are less so, thank her for helping you gather more data before making major decisions and not jumping to conclusions so easily.

If she's intuitive and perceptive, and you take things at face value, thank her for helping you read between the lines and learning that some things are not black and white but have a deeper meaning upon close inspection.

If she does things at a slower pace than you, thank her for making you "stop and smell the roses."

If she's more family oriented than you, thank her for providing you with security, comfort, loyalty, and devotion.

If she has a lively sense of humor, thank her for making you laugh and lightening your burdens.

If she shares her good fortune with others and is a giver, thank her for teaching you not to be so selfish and possessive.

If she's less worried about the future than you are, tell her you appreciate her for making you enjoy the present.

If she believes in you more than you believe in yourself, thank her for giving you more confidence in your abilities and helping you strive for more.

If she's ambitious, thank her for helping you strive for more and not settling for less than is attainable.

Tell her that who she is, her basic core, is what you adore and appreciate about her with all your heart. Make her feel that she matters to you, that she has made a difference in your life, and that without her, you could not be as happy or satisfied as you have become.

Do you see how important it is to have someone who is so different from you? Her strengths are usually your weaknesses, and your strengths will usually turn out to be what she needs to grow as a person.

## WHY A WOMAN FALLS IN LOVE

A woman falls in love because of the way she feels about herself when she's with you. The majority of women I've studied have said that they felt prettier, sexier, more intelligent, more capable, and more needed when that special man came into their lives than they ever felt about themselves before.

Geri summed it up when she said, "When I fell in love, I felt perfect, as if I could do no wrong. For the first time, someone loved me for who I was, and that was a glorious feeling."

Don't destroy the glow you found when she first fell in love with you.

Carol explained, "My father was not a complimentary-type person. He used to tell me I had big ears and no breasts and that it should be the other way around. Needless to say, I didn't grow up feeling very attractive. Then Matthew came along and told me how he loved my sexy legs, soft skin, and beautiful smile. He used to say that wherever I was, I lit up the place. I find that I walk a little taller and am more self-assured because of my wonderful husband."

Martha said she had felt stupid most of her life because she was always a bit slower than her brothers and sisters. "Ted made me feel I was a capable human being. Every time I started putting myself down, he made me stop and rephrase what I had to say, leaving out the part where I belittled myself. Over and over he told me how wonderful and smart I was. He actually convinced me that I had more going for me than I thought."

Jo grew up with alcoholic parents. Her father became

verbally abusive and sometimes abused her physically as well. She recalled, "Bruce came over one night to pick me up, and my father was already drunk by the time he got there. He was swearing and throwing things. Bruce walked over to him, looked him right in the eye, and said, 'If you say or do one more thing to Jo, I'm going to deck you!' Right then and there, I knew I wanted to spend the rest of my life with this man. He was my knight in shining armor. After thirty-three years, I still feel the same way. He's never stopped protecting me."

Bonnie fell in love with Roger, her boss. She was his executive secretary. "When I first came to work for him, his office was a shambles. I reorganized and rearranged everything. Soon he was taking me with him to all his business meetings and even began asking my opinion on some deals on which he was working. He really respected me, and I enjoyed the feeling because it was mutual. We've been married for eleven years, and I love the feeling of being needed. He still consults me before making any final decisions."

Ever since she could remember, Tina wanted to help people who were less fortunate than she. She came from a wealthy family and was expected to act like a respectable member of that family. When she announced she was joining the Peace Corps, her family was shocked. "It was there that I met my husband, Ned. He, too, was very young and idealistic, but we had the same dream. He understood me, and I loved being with someone who shared the same goals as I did. Today we have six adopted handicapped children and couldn't be happier. My parents hardly speak to me anymore."

Marla took her turn. "I had cancer and had to have one of my breasts removed. I was only thirty-two at the time and felt I would never find a man who could love me. Kent and I started dating, and when the inevitable day came, I felt compelled to tell him. He took me in his arms and said, 'Don't you think you mean more to me than that?' We got married, and I can honestly say I feel sexy in spite of what happened. It's all because of my kind, gentle, loving husband."

These women all have very special men in their lives who have boosted their self-esteem. No wonder they are so full of praise and respect for them.

## SHE'S WORTH EIGHT COWS

Many years ago I read a story that I have never been able to forget. It was called "The Eight Cow Wife." It's about a Polynesian boy, Johnny Lingo, who fell in love with a young girl on a nearby island. The girl had been degraded by her father until she had no self-esteem left. In this particular society, when you wanted to get married, you bartered with cows. If the girl was very plain and ordinary, you could pay her father one cow. If she was an exceptional woman, you might wind up giving three or four cows. Women took great personal pride in the number of cows needed for the trade. Johnny could have easily traded one cow for this young girl, and her father would have been thrilled just to get rid of her. Instead, Johnny offered eight cows, which shocked the whole village. When asked why he gave so many, he said he wanted everyone, especially his new wife, to know how much he felt she was worth. Later, when one of the townspeople came to call on Johnny Lingo, he could not believe his eyes when he saw Johnny's wife. She had changed from an ugly young girl into one of the most beautiful young women he had ever seen.

Low self-esteem is one of the most common reasons for depression in women. If you treat a woman like a thoroughbred, you won't have a nag. If you put a high value on the woman in your life, I guarantee she will try her best to be worthy of your appreciation. If people think highly of you, then you don't want to disappoint them. You have a natural tendency to try to live up to their expectations. On the other hand, if they degrade you, there's nothing to strive for.

It takes a tremendous amount of love and tenderness to bring out the best in a woman.

In the film *Seven Beauties,* the main character, played by Giancarlo Giannini, says, "Every woman has a sweetness somewhere inside her. She may seem bitter on the outside, like a cup of coffee when the sugar has settled to the bottom. She needs stirring to bring the sugar to your lips."

## A FATHER'S APPROVAL

I grew up being a "daddy's girl." My father always used that term to describe me. He came from Europe and was a baker by trade. Working full time during the day and part time at night, he had little time left to do anything but sleep. And yet I remember the precious time we did spend together; he always showered me with praise and affection. He used to sit me on his lap and sing, "You Are My Sunshine." When I was eight, he took the whole family to the Catskill Mountains. My brother and I were allowed to go to the hotel's nightclub with our parents. As the band played, my father asked me to dance. Everyone started clapping and making a circle around us, and he swung me in his arms and over his back. Even though I was only eight years old, it's still a vivid memory.

It wasn't until I researched material for the men's class that I realized what significance my upbringing had for me. Male approval is so important to a woman. A woman's father is the first man in her life that either gives or withholds it. I had so much approval growing up that my husband didn't need to supply me with a tremendous amount. Yet many women did not have such a loving, doting father. They spend the rest of their lives looking for approval they never got. Yes, you have to fill the gap. If you don't, she'll keep looking until she finds it. It's not something she can live without.

So here's your choice.

You can concentrate on who she's not, what she hasn't accomplished, what she's not capable of doing, what she's always doing incorrectly, how inferior she is, and how she just doesn't measure up to your expectations. If that's the path you choose, your payoff will be a cold, bitter, cynical, frightened, unresponsive woman.

If you choose to concentrate on loving her for who she is, appreciating her strengths, noticing the little things she does, praising her for the small accomplishments, reinforcing her capabilities, and raising her value as a human being, your payoff will be a woman who worships the ground you walk on, caters to your needs, responds to you passionately, and will never want to live without you.

## ACTION ASSIGNMENT #1

What? Homework assignments? Absolutely! What good is reading all this without my leading your knowledge to action? The only way new behavior can become part of you is to practice, see the results, and find out for yourself what a wonderful effect it has on your mate. Yes, this will take time and effort, but you'll be rewarded with a loving, understanding, passionate woman who will be more responsive to you and, in turn, will take more of her time and effort to fulfill your needs.

Let's get started, and watch her respond to your new loving behavior! Invest in some index cards on which you can copy the assignments and have constant reminders at your fingertips. Most of us spend a great deal of time in our cars or on public transit getting to and from work. Make good use of this time (of course, if you're in a car, do it only at stop lights). Keep these cards in your briefcase or lunchbox or glove compartment, and every so often take them out and read them. This way, the new behavior will become a permanent part of your life.

1. Make sure that at least once this week you tell her that who she is, her basic core, is what you adore.
2. Take her in your arms and tell her how much value she has as a human being.
3. Look at the lists in this chapter to see which of her traits you have been trying to change and try to view them in a positive light. Let her know what you like about her personality. Reinforce her capabilities.
4. Notice the little things she does for you and tell her that you appreciate them.

Dear Ellen,

I just had to write and tell you what happened last Friday, because I know you'll get a kick out of it. While at an office party that spouses were invited to, I was ranting and raving about your class to Willis, one of Gary's co-workers. You can't imagine the look on his face when I began talking about some of the changes that have taken place in Gary and in our twenty-six-year marriage. When I was done, Willis said with a sigh of relief, "The whole office thinks that Gary is having an affair. We've been hearing him whispering and laughing on the phone, seeing him ordering flowers and candy, and watching him leave for extended lunches." They had no idea that the affair Gary was having was with me! We've been having these afternoon rendezvous ever since he took your class.

Thanks for contributing to office gossip!

Love,

Jeanette

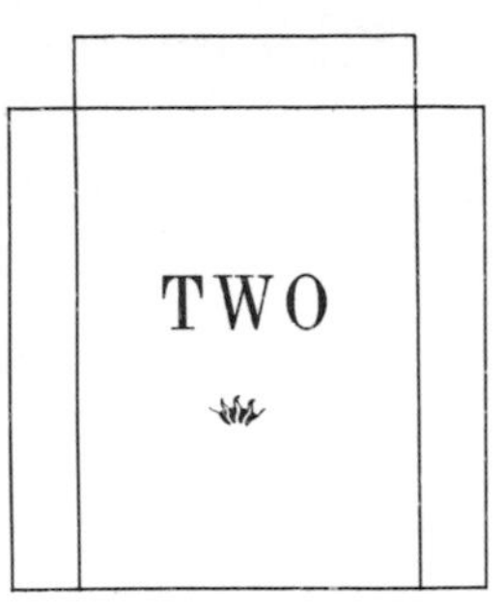

# From Her Point of View

## WHO CAN UNDERSTAND A WOMAN?

Ask a man what the perfect woman would be like, and often he will say, "I want her to be a lady during the day and a mistress at night." Ask that same man what he thinks a woman wants in a man, and his response most often is, "You've got me. Who can understand them? They're too complicated. She doesn't know what she wants!"

Henry Higgins, in *My Fair Lady,* could not understand Eliza, so he asked, "Why can't a woman be more like a man?" Why can't a woman be more like a man, indeed. She can't be like a man because she is decidedly different from a man. This frustration is shared by many men who wish it weren't so.

A wonderful place to begin to unravel the mystery, to begin to understand the complexity of a woman's needs, is the following list:

- She wants to be your first priority.
- She wants you to consider her needs above everyone else's.

- She wants you to think that no other woman comes close to being as wonderful for you as she is.
- She wants you to brag about her to your friends and family.
- She wants you to feel proud that she's your mate.
- She wants you to prove your love.
- She wants you to think she's the most beautiful woman alive.
- She wants you to think that who she is and what she does is nothing short of miraculous.
- She wants tender, loving care at that special time every month when her emotions are ruled by her hormones.
- She needs and expects to have daily reminders of how much you love her.

From her point of view, she needs to believe that you are constantly thinking of her and that you are counting the moments until she will be in your arms again. This may be only a fantasy for her, but with a little effort from you, it can come true. You, too, can join the ranks of great lovers, those men who are able to turn a woman's fantasy into reality.

## WHAT DO WOMEN WANT?

She wants to be at the top of your list of priorities. She wants the number one position. She wants to mean more to you than your friends and co-workers, your clients, your secretary, or even your mother.

She constantly compares the amount of time you spend with her to the amount of time you spend with other people or activities.

She constantly compares the amount of energy you have with her to the amount of energy you have with other people.

She constantly compares the amount of respect you have for her feelings to the amount of respect you have for other people's feelings.

Bill volunteered that he was so involved with activities outside the home that Lois hardly ever saw him. He sat on every committee the community offered. "I am an insurance agent, and the only way I can build my business is to make as many contacts with people as I can," he said in defense of his actions.

I explained that unless he wanted to become a successful *divorced* insurance agent, he'd better spend some quality time with his wife; he'd have to find a balance between his desire for success and his love for her. What he didn't know at the time he enrolled in my class was that Lois was beginning to think about having an affair with someone in her exercise class.

She had confided in me, "I am so lonely. Bill is just never there, and along comes Tom, who I see at least three times a week. We've gone out for coffee twice, and I find I'm really attracted to him."

Soon after Bill took "Light Her Fire," Lois had changed gyms, and she and Bill were in an aerobics class together.

Milton finally understood why Maureen was constantly complaining. "I usually come home exhausted from work and became a couch potato. If Maureen asked me to do her a favor, I was usually too tired and found some excuse not to help her. But if a neighbor or friend stopped by, I always had the strength to talk and laugh and have a few beers. I somehow found the energy to go out drinking with my buddies on Friday night, but not to take my wife out on Saturday night. I realize now how unfair I've been. Maureen deserves more than I have been giving. I was spending quality time with everyone except the woman I love."

Jack explained the hostility his wife felt toward his mother. "I'll admit that my mother is a very controlling woman. She expects me to jump whenever she says so. It's always been that way. I'm her oldest son, and somehow I feel responsible for her. No matter what time, day or night, when she wants something, I usually drop what I'm doing so I can take care of whatever she needs. I am ashamed to say that one time when my wife and I were making love, my mother called, telling me that her kitchen sink was stopped up. Instead of saying, 'I'll call you back'—or better yet, not answering the phone in the first place—I sat there yessing her to death and ended up telling her I'd be there in about half an hour. Instead of telling her to call a plumber, I put her needs ahead of my wife's needs."

My husband began doing a wonderful thing years ago and still does it to this day. He always tells his secretary, "I am not to be disturbed when I'm in a meeting; the only exception is my wife. No matter what I'm in the middle of, if she calls, let her through." Now, do I feel important, special, and loved? You bet I do! I'm more important to him than anyone else in this whole world. By the way, he is always glad to hear from me, and I don't ever feel that

I'm an annoyance he wants to get rid of. He always takes the time to listen to what I have to say.

Many men act cold and indifferent on the phone when their mates call them at work, as if to say, "How dare you call? This had better be important. I have more pressing issues than to listen to your problems right now." It's no wonder this type of man returns home at night to a cold, bitter woman.

She constantly wants your love validated. It's almost as if she is forever asking, Who do you love more?

Your job or me?
Your friends or me?
Your mother or me?
Your children or me?
This house or me?
Your freedom or me?
Your hobby or me?
Your clients or me?

Nate, who was separated from Marie, said, "I never made her feel like she mattered. I had my priorities really mixed up. I put my job first, then my friends, next my family, and Marie was last. I went out of my way to make everyone else feel special, and felt that 'good ol' Marie' would always be there for me. Well, she wasn't, and now I'm going to put her first and see if I can win her back."

By the fourth class he had accomplished his goal, and he said that things were better for both him and Marie than they'd ever been before. Nate had finally learned that you can never take your relationship for granted.

## THERE'S NO COMPARISON

Don't ever compare your mate to another woman, especially your mother, your ex-wife, or some dear old girlfriend. This is a major cause of hurt for many women. If you have one or two favorite recipes that your mother cooked, by all means let her pass them on. But that's where it has to stop. On the same note, never talk wistfully about other relationships you may have had. While these relationships might be long over in your own mind, for her, the comparison will be obvious. Don't expect her to understand, because she probably won't. You'll only create insecurity where there should be none.

A man who wants to re-create the past is headed for trouble. Remember, she wants to be number one in your life. It's very hard to feel that way when given a role model—your mother, your ex-wife, or some old flame—she believes she has to follow.

Conrad confessed that his wife was furious just after Christmas. "Looking back, I can understand why. I had the nerve to give Bernice an entire cookbook of my mother's recipes. I even went to the trouble of labeling the holiday dinners with stars. At the time, I couldn't understand why Bernice cried for three days. After what I've learned in 'Light Her Fire,' I now see how awful my wife must have felt. My mother was a full-time housewife and a gourmet cook. Bernice works eight hours a day and can hardly get through the door at night. The last thing she wants to do is cook a gourmet meal when she gets home. Just this week, I threw the cookbook away. I apologized to Bernice and told her that I would never compare her to my mother again. After all, Bernice has so many strengths of her own. Why should I want her to be something she's not?"

David made the big mistake of comparing Sharon to their next-door neighbor, Darla. He had gone out drinking with Eddie, Darla's husband, and as the evening progressed, they began talking about matters better kept to themselves. Eddie told David how many times a week he and Darla had sex and how Darla never turned him down. David came back home and in a kidding way said to Sharon, "I should be moving in one house down—lucky guy!" Sharon was so hurt, she started screaming, "Why don't you? I thought we had something special, and now you go blabbing our personal life to the neighbors and compare me to that sickly woman who spends more time at the doctor's office than at home. She's nothing but a hypochondriac, and you deserve each other!"

I didn't want to guess how long it would be before David got out of the doghouse for that one.

Amy explained she had a wonderful career when she married Rick, and that was one of the things he admired most about her. But when they came back from their honeymoon, Rick's mother gave her a list of everyone in the family to whom she was expected to send Christmas cards. She told the class, "When I saw the sixty-five names and addresses of his aunts, uncles, cousins, etc., I almost cried. When I tried to explain to Rick that I never send cards even to my own family, that this was overwhelming to me, he couldn't understand why. After all, his mother always did this, so what was the big deal? I told him I wasn't his mother."

Every woman wants to be admired for her own strengths

and not be compared to any other woman you know. Treat her as though she is truly the number one woman in your life, allow her to be the competent woman she really is, and you will be surprised how quickly she will adapt to that role.

## WHAT A DIFFERENCE A FRIEND MAKES

I've heard women say many times, "He acts so differently toward me when he's around his friends than when we're alone together." Some men feel the need to project a "macho" image with their friends. They don't want to appear dependent or serious about their mate, so they go out of their way to act independent and carefree. They won't hold hands, put an arm around her, or exhibit any behavior that demonstrates how much they love her. What a mistake not to show everyone, including your mate, how much you love her and how important she is in your life.

Joe admitted the difference in his behavior when he was alone with his wife and when he was with his friends. "When Agnes and I are alone, I'm very attentive and loving. But it's true, when my friends come over, I change completely. If Agnes says something, I tend to ignore her and go right on talking as if she didn't exist. Sometimes I've even pretended I didn't hear her or rolled my eyes as if to say, 'Can you believe her?' We always wind up having an argument after they leave."

Catherine said, "I don't stay around when Mike's friends come over, because I used to get so angry. Whenever he started talking, he'd drop the word 'we' and only use 'I,' as if I were not even in his life. If I tried to participate in the conversation, he'd make some sarcastic remark. It would take me at least two days to forgive him. So now, I just leave."

Mary said that one night she and her husband were walking, his arm around her shoulder, her arm around his waist. When two of his friends came toward them, he dropped her like a hot potato. "I was shocked at how awkward and uncomfortable he seemed standing next to me and talking to them. When they left, I questioned him about this, and he said, 'They don't have girlfriends, so they wouldn't understand.' 'Understand what?' I asked. 'That we're in love? You don't think they would understand that?' I was livid!"

The message that this kind of behavior sends to a woman is:

- He's embarrassed about me.
- He really doesn't care about me.
- His friends are more important than I am.

The message you always want to send is:

- I'm so proud to be with you.
- I really care about you.
- You are the most important person in my life.

## PROVE YOUR LOVE

Women want you to prove your love in some tangible way. Love really does have to be verbalized and demonstrated every day in small ways. You have to walk up to the plate before you can hit a home run. Many times she'll ask you to do her a favor, like rubbing her back, getting her a glass of water, stopping by the store on your way home from work, getting her a towel, answering the phone, or calling her when you get to your destination. When you respond to her request without objections or excuses, she thinks, *He loves me.* On the other hand, if you respond with, "I'm too tired, it's too far, I'm too busy," she thinks, *He doesn't love me.*

So the next time she makes a request, *grant it.* Remember, proving your love always involves extra time, money, or effort spent in making her feel special.

## LITTLE THINGS MEAN A LOT

I was in a cab when the driver and I began conversing. I told him I was working on this book, and he said, "Well, I know what women want—to have a lot of money spent on them."

How wrong he was. A woman is capable of spending a lot of money all by herself. She's perfectly capable of picking out a new washer and dryer or a table and lamp. She needs you to prove your love with romantic gifts that are personal, gifts that show her that you are willing to spend time and effort solely on her. Just in case you haven't been told yet, a fishing rod, a toolbox, a lawn mower, a chain saw, or camping equipment do not qualify as romantic gifts.

The following are just some examples of what women love to receive.

- Flowers—The supermarket provides them inexpensively
- Cards—romantic, not funny ones, please
- A letter you wrote all by yourself
- Jewelry
- Perfume
- A music box
- An outfit she's wanted
- A nightgown
- Chocolate candy
- A beautiful vase
- A plaque with a romantic poem on it
- A ceramic figure that has special meaning
- A stuffed animal
- An overnight stay at a hotel
- A book of poetry

It can be challenging and fun to buy a small, inexpensive gift and present it in an imaginative way. After this class, many men, eager to prove their love, became very creative.

Gerald told us, "My wife, Kay, eats Total cereal for breakfast every morning, so I went to the supermarket and got a box of Special K. I wrapped the two boxes of cereal together, tied them with a big bow, and left a note, 'To my Special K, the most complete and Total woman I know.' I can tell you, my homecoming that night was very special. Such a little thing meant so much to her."

Chip bought a box of Good and Plenty candy and put it in his wife's purse. He added a note that said, "To my wonderful wife, who gives me Good and Plenty love." She called him as soon as she arrived at work to tell him that he had made her day.

Rusty leaves for work very early in the morning. The night before, he went to a florist and got one rose and one violet. The next morning, he put them both on his pillow next to his sleeping wife with a note, "Roses are red, violets are blue. Even though I'm at work, I'm thinking of you." That night, he was treated like a king. "I always thought you needed a lot of money to please a woman," he said, "but I've learned that just two flowers can be as effective as a fur coat."

Cecil bought a small ceramic eagle and attached a note that said, "I can fly higher than an eagle with you by my side," then left it on the vanity, where his wife was sure to find it. That eagle is now one of her most treasured possessions.

All these men were surprised at how imaginative and creative they could be when they put their minds to it. The gifts they gave may have been small, but the resulting appreciation was priceless.

Whatever you decide to give her, be sure that it is a complete gift. Always do a little extra. If it is a vase, put flowers in it. If it is a music box, put a little note in it. If it can be wrapped, wrap it. Women love opening packages. And whatever you do, if it is a candy dish, put candy in it.

Even after twenty-four years of marriage, I still remember our first Valentine's Day. My husband had forgotten. At first I thought he was kidding, but he was serious. I cried the entire day. Finally, at around eight o'clock that night, he ran to a store and grabbed a candy dish and brought it home. When I saw the dish I cried even harder, because I knew no thought had gone into its purchase at all. I was on a diet, and he had bought a candy dish! (He didn't even have the sense to put candy in it!)

My husband did not come from a family that bought presents. He never saw his father bring his mother flowers, so he really didn't think that birthdays or anniversaries were any big deal. Well, to me they were. It's a day when you take time to prove your love. To me and many other women, the gift says, "You are worthwhile." Not giving a gift is saying, "You are worthless."

I could have tried to intellectualize the situation and take the rational approach: a) I knew his background; b) I know he loves me; and c) I know I really matter to him, with or without a gift. I tried to do that, but I was overruled by my emotions and wound up hurt, angry, and disappointed. I must have remained cold and distant for at least a week, but then I melted as he took me in his arms and said, "I promise I'll never forget Valentine's Day again." He's kept his promise, and I love him all the more for it.

There are five holidays you should never forget, and on those special days be sure to give her something that is a little more extravagant. A man who forgets any of these special days will devastate his woman. Here are the Special Dates.

*Her Birthday*—Always buy her something personal that you think she'd like, or something she's been asking for. One of the men in my class always sent a thank-you card to her parents on his wife's birthday. He'd always write about how grateful he was to them for having her. Now, that's a thoughtful man. Her parents, by the way, think he's the greatest husband on earth and he can do no wrong in their eyes.

*Your Anniversary*—A card is a must. A letter along with the card telling her what she means to you is extra proof of your devotion. On this occasion, it's appropriate to plan a getaway. All arrangements, including the baby-sitter, should be handled by you.

*Valentine's Day*—A card and a box of candy or a special arrangement of flowers say, "You are my sweetheart."

*Christmas or Hanukkah*—This is when every store is filled with gift suggestions, and the salespeople are very helpful. During this holiday season, every Sunday paper has a pull-out supplement on gift ideas. There's no excuse for lack of imagination here.

*Mother's Day*—There are two gifts you need to get on this day. The first is for your mother. If you've assigned this task to your wife, please take it back and assume full responsibility. There's nothing more insulting for a mother than to get a card signed by her daughter-in-law for you. Your wife can buy her a mother-in-law card on her own, but don't give her the burden of taking care of this holiday. Although your wife may not be aware of it, a resentment builds year after year when she is responsible for your obligations.

The second gift, of course, is for your wife, the mother of your child. There's such great pleasure for a woman whose husband starts this ritual when the child is born. When the toddler marches over to Mommy with her present, and then you give her yours, there's hardly a woman I know who doesn't get teary-eyed. When children reach school age, you no longer have to worry about her getting a present from them. Every teacher dedicates a few hours of art class to creating a special gift for Mom. What mother doesn't delight in displaying that clay object or picture made for her by the hands of her little one? And what woman doesn't delight in having a husband who appreciates what a wonderful mother she is and proves with a gift just how lucky his children are to have a mother like her?

Another event that is appropriate for gift giving is the birth of your child. A woman has just gone through nine months of pregnancy, hard work in itself. She deserves a present that says, "I'm so thankful for this miracle we brought into our lives." Jewelry, like a bracelet or a pendant with a baby charm attached and engraved, would be wonderful. A comfortable nightgown to wear in the hospital would also be welcomed.

While we're on the subject of hospitals, anytime your girlfriend or wife is recuperating from surgery and has to stay in the hospital for any reason, a gift is definitely appropriate and appreciated.

To this day, I remember the flower arrangement my husband sent to my hospital room after I had surgery. The beauty and fragrance of those flowers brought me hours of pleasure. There's not much else you can do but stare when you've had an operation, and there's nothing more depressing than a sterile hospital room. So the flowers my husband sent were a welcome addition. All the nurses came in and commented about what a gorgeous arrangement it was. One nurse said, "Boy, you sure have someone who loves you." How secure and happy that made me feel, two good feelings that helped speed my recovery time.

If your mate is sick at home, little things mean a lot. Matt, a young man in his twenties, wanted to do something for his girlfriend after hearing my lecture on gift giving. She was home from work, recovering from a ski accident. Here's what I recommended.

A phone call at least twice a day.

A box of candy.

Some of her favorite magazines.

Cassette tapes to listen to. He bought some motivational tapes as well as music.

Comedy videos. You can buy or rent them at your neighborhood video store.

Pretty stationery, so she could write some letters to friends. He also included a beautiful pen and stamps.

Was he her hero! She never stopped telling her friends what a special man he was and how lucky she was to have him. I'd say that's a pretty good return on his investment.

## PICK IT OUT YOURSELF

Whatever the occasion, please buy the gift yourself. I know there are many shopping services, including secretaries, that can do your shopping for you, but if your mate finds out that it wasn't from you, she'll be very hurt.

Saul told the following story. "For me, money is not a problem, but time is. I'm a surgeon, and I'm always very busy. For my wife's birthday one year, I decided to use a shopping service. The service chose a ring, which they could get at a good price, and told me that it would be a very personal, appropriate gift. I agreed. My wife was overjoyed when she opened her present, and she wore it all the time and showed it to all her friends. Six months later she went to a luncheon, and the woman next to her had on the same ring. When I came home that night, she told me with tears in her eyes what the woman had said: 'I guess our husbands subscribe to the same shopping service. That's where all my gifts come from.' My wife has never put that ring on again, and I have learned a valuable lesson. The time and thought I put into selecting a gift for her means more than the gift itself. I'll never hurt her feelings that way again."

As a result of my class on giving, Tyrone now has the confidence to buy gifts for his wife by himself, even the intimate kind. "I've always wanted to buy my wife a negligee, but I was too embarrassed to go into the lingerie department. After Ellen described how much fun this could be despite any embarrassment I might feel, I finally decided to do it. I went to a department store that was quite some distance from home so I wouldn't be recognized (I still wasn't *that* brave yet!), parked the car, took a deep breath, and repeated over and over, 'This can be fun, and it will mean a lot to my wife.' The saleslady was so helpful, and when I finally decided on the negligee I wanted, she looked at me and said, 'Your wife is really lucky to have a man like you. My husband would never do this.' The woman in the gift-wrapping department was impressed too. She nodded her head and said, 'She sure is a lucky woman.' I walked out proud of myself, full of a new feeling of confidence.

"My wife was blown away when she opened the package. She immediately put the negligee on and began modeling it for me. We had a wonderful afternoon. That negligee is only the beginning of a whole new intimate wardrobe my wife is going to get."

## SAY SOMETHING, NOTICE EVERYTHING

After twenty-four years of marriage, Doris wanted a divorce. Her husband, Greg, was shocked when she told him, and he sat there with a dumbfounded look and asked, "Why?"

He told about her answer. "Doris walked over to me, covered my eyes with her hands, and asked me, 'What color are the flowers on the kitchen wallpaper?' My initial response was, 'Are you nuts? How should I know? What does this have to do with you wanting a divorce?' When she left the room in disgust, I started thinking. I had lived in that house for nine years, and inconceivable as it was, I really didn't know what color those flowers were. I was completely oblivious to most things that didn't involve my job. At work, I paid attention to every little detail. Not only had I stopped noticing my own home, but somewhere during the years I had stopped noticing my wife."

Noticing a woman makes her feel alive. It makes her feel as if she matters to you. When she feels as if she's invisible, a little part of the love she felt in the beginning dies.

When this kind of situation arises, many men feel that they've said nothing to upset their mate and can't understand why she's being distant or angry. The reason she's acting that way is because you've said *nothing* and noticed *nothing* when she has made changes, gone out of her way to look pretty, or gone to some extra effort to please you.

Serena agreed with many of the women who shared the same concerns one evening. "Marlin never notices when I've gone to the beauty parlor. I could be bald, and I don't think he'd know the difference."

Paula added, "Ted never comments on how I look, even when we get dressed up to go somewhere."

Sandy complained that even when she cooks a special meal, she never gets a compliment.

Someone in one of my classes handed me a wonderful quote from Alberto Giacometti, the twentieth-century sculptor. "To look at the same face every day of the year and never fail to find something new in it is the greatest of adventures and greater by far than any journey 'round the world."

You have to make a conscious decision to notice the woman in your life, then verbalize your approval or admiration with a compliment. If you're thinking that she already knows you like the way she looks, the way she cooks, or that you're proud of her, it's not enough. *It has to be verbalized.* Saying nothing is always taken as an insult, never a compliment.

When a woman has to ask you how she looks, she's already thinking, "He doesn't think I look good," or she is hurt that you didn't notice. If she has to ask if you liked the dinner, she's already thinking, "He doesn't like it," or she is annoyed that you didn't notice that she went to a lot of trouble to please you.

Don't let a day go by without taking time out to notice that wonderful woman. Compliment her every day on something she's done, who she is, or on her physical appearance.

## THE FIVE-SECOND COMPLIMENT

Many men have said that they never saw their father give their mother a compliment, nor did they get any themselves. I know it's always difficult to give what you didn't get yourself, but you need to make a conscious decision to do it anyway, because it means so much to her.

Ryan said, "It's not that I don't think nice things. I just don't take the time to say them."

Robert said, "I really don't know what to say so that it doesn't sound phony."

In my workshop, I teach men how to give a compliment. For some of you this may be elementary, but believe me, many men simply haven't learned what a woman wants to hear. In giving a compliment, you have to be descriptive and specific. Generalities are appropriate for strangers but not for the most important person in your life. This will take a little practice, but I know you'll get the hang of it once you've done it a few times. What you get in return will be worth your extra effort. Sometimes a five-second compliment makes her feel wonderful for four hours. All you need to do is be more generous with the words you give her.

General statement:

- You look nice.

Change that to:

- Wow, that red dress really looks beautiful on you. It shows off your fantastic figure.

Or:

- You look so pretty in pink. It makes your skin glow.
- I love the length of that dress. It shows off your sexy legs.
- You are a knockout in that outfit. Every man at that party is going to envy me.

General Statement:

- The dinner was good.

Change that to:

- Honey, that dinner was wonderful. The mashed potatoes were so creamy, and the roast was delicious.

Or:

- This is the best fried chicken I've ever tasted. There's not a restaurant anywhere that can compare to your cooking.
- Thank you so much for going to all that trouble tonight. The meal was terrific. I'm the luckiest man alive to have such a wonderful cook for a wife.

General statement:

- I love sex.

Change that to:

- You are so sexy. You really turn me on.

Or:

- You are the most exciting woman alive. I'm so lucky to have you.
- I feel so complete, having a woman like you by my side.
- You take my breath away. You are the most wonderful lover a man could have.
- Holding you in my arms is the closest thing to heaven. You feel so good.

My point here is that when you take a little more time to give her a more complete compliment, you will have a woman who feels more complete. When she asks if you love her, and your reply is "Yup," think of how much more meaningful it would be to say, "I love you more than life itself. I can't imagine ever living without you. You mean everything to me."

The week following my presentation on the art of complimenting, Wayne came to class thrilled by his new ability. He explained that he and his wife, Becky, had planned a weekend away together. When they left on Friday evening, Becky was exhausted and depressed. She had just spent the week at home nursing their son through the flu, her dad was recovering from surgery, and her best friend was getting divorced. Wayne said that had he not taken the class, he would have gotten angry at her for ruining the trip with her "poor me" attitude. "Instead," he said, "I pulled over to the side of the road, stopped the engine, and bombarded her with compliments. I told her that our children were the luckiest kids in the world to have a mom like her, her parents were lucky to have such a caring, loving daughter, and I was the luckiest man alive to have such a wonderful wife. I told her she was beautiful and intelligent. I went on complimenting her for about ten minutes." He told the other men in the room that for those ten minutes he gave her, he got back a woman who provided him with hours of enjoyment. "We both were able to focus on each other for the entire weekend," he said, beaming.

Some other things that you should be extra sensitive to are:

- A woman's fear of getting older and less attractive to you. When she shows you a new wrinkle or line on her face, she'd love to hear how she looks more beautiful with every year that passes.
- If she's trying to better herself by going back to school or learning a new skill, she'd love to hear how much you admire her.
- If she's trying to overcome a problem like overeating or smoking, she'd love to hear how special she is for trying to improve herself.

In other words, every chance you get, build her up. Don't ever tear her down. Why? Because a woman who feels good about herself when she's with you is automatically motivated to satisfy your needs, care about your feelings, and will try to please you. In the end, you'll experience more harmony in your life.

## ONE WEEK OF GIVING

It's impossible, even for the most oblivious man, not to notice that each month his mate exhibits some strange behavior that doesn't seem to occur the rest of the time. When I asked men in my classes what they've observed in this context, the following were common responses.

"It's like clockwork. She goes berserk for a few days, then returns to normal."

"Let's put it this way. If she had acted on our first date like she does every time she's about to menstruate, there wouldn't have been a second date."

"My wife overreacts to anything I say. It's the only time she accuses me of not loving her."

"She becomes so irrational; I can't deal with her."

"I know when it's coming, because she cries a lot."

"She can't cope with life."

"She drives me nuts."

One night in class, Reed asked me if I knew the difference between a woman with PMS and a terrorist. When I said no, he smiled and said, "You can negotiate with a terrorist."

Can you imagine feeling just wonderful one day, feeling that everything in your life is working, that you have no worries or problems to solve, and then, all of a sudden, you get a migraine headache and can hardly see, your stomach gets bloated, and you are physically exhausted to the point of hardly being able to get out of bed? Add dizziness, cramps, and nausea to that, and you'll begin to have some idea of what a woman goes through every month. What I've just described is PMS, Premenstrual Syndrome. It has not been labeled "the curse" for no reason.

As difficult as she may be, these are the times she needs extra love, extra tenderness, extra understanding, and extra care from you. Your turn will come someday, when you are simply feeling under the weather due to a cold, flu, or high blood pressure. If you'll learn to baby her during these times of extreme stress, she will do the same for you. On the other hand, if you ignore her, or worse, say something like, "I'll stay away, you're obviously on the rag," she'll never forget, and you'll get yours! She has a memory like an elephant.

Whether you are with your present mate or exchange her for someone else, you are still going to get a *woman.* Every month, for at least one week, she will experience these symptoms to some degree. The slightest things you say or do can trigger overreaction and cause her great emotional upset.

Here are the things I suggest you do.

Offer to cook dinner, take her to a restaurant, or get takeout food and bring it home.

Be extra abundant with compliments and appreciation.

Offer to take her to the movies, or rent movies and allow her to "vegetate."

Don't make any extra requests during that week. Make those phone calls and run those errands yourself.

Go out of your way to be extra helpful with the children. Offer to baby-sit and encourage her to do what she wants, whether it be shopping or relaxing in the tub.

A loving relationship means that sometimes you give a hundred percent of yourself and you may get back very little at that moment. But the tables will turn. All of a sudden you may find that you have nothing to give, and lo and behold, she's the one who's giving you a hundred percent. That's how we balance each other.

I remember my mother waiting on my father hand and foot, catering to his every whim. My brother and I had gotten married, so all the attention she used to give us now went to my father. Prior to her death a few years ago, I saw firsthand how her giving was being repaid. She had heart trouble and was extremely tired most of the time. I was very surprised to see my father taking care of all her needs. He would get her medication or a glass of water, serve her dinner, clean up the dishes, help her get dressed, and do everything he could to see that she was comfortable.

When I commented on how nice it was, he said, "I figure it this way. She babied me for many years; now it's my turn."

Since then, there has never been any doubt in my mind as to how much my father loved my mother.

Maurice was a delightful man in his late sixties who took the men's course for enjoyment. He and Mabel had been married for forty-eight years. He shared with the class that "Mabel's time of the month usually lasted two weeks, and we made a pact early on in our marriage. We agreed that since there were four weeks to every month, I'd be in charge of most things for two weeks, and she'd take control again for the other two weeks." We all laughed when he added, "Of course, I couldn't wait for the two weeks when she felt good again. I didn't like doing the laundry, food shopping, and dishes, but I did it anyway."

The give and take is what makes a relationship so rewarding. Even though it may not seem so at times, you will always get back what you give. To give love and be loved are the most precious gifts in life and should be cherished above all else.

## VERBALIZE YOUR LOVE

Many men don't say "I love you" very frequently, or they don't say it at all, because they're thinking, "She knows I love her. Why do I have to tell her?" A woman needs to hear "I love you" at least three times a day. Usually when I've made this statement, men and women who have been happily married for many years agree immediately.

Herb said, "I've been married for forty-three years and can't imagine leaving in the morning without kissing Bess and saying 'I love you' and certainly at night before we go to sleep. We also speak on the phone several times a day and always end with 'I love you.' "

Howard, who was about to be married, said, "I can't even count how many times a day we say 'I love you.' "

Lowell said that Karen finally broke up with him because he never said "I love you." "It used to drive her crazy. I always told her that it was difficult for me, because I came from a family who never said they cared, but that was really no excuse. Now I wish I had another chance."

Too many people use their past as an excuse for ruining the present. You have to make a conscious decision to love someone in a way that you know makes that person feel good. It may not be important to you, or it may be difficult for you, but if the woman in your life needs to hear those words, and such a simple request is denied, then she thinks,

"Do I really want to spend the rest of my life with someone who makes me feel so empty?"

Tell her, over and over, again and again, those three little words that mean so much to her: "I love you." She'll never get tired of hearing them.

## ACTION ASSIGNMENT #2

1. Write her a love letter this week. Tell her how much she means to you. Review some wonderful moments you've shared with her. Send it through the mail; it's more romantic that way.
2. Praise her in front of someone else once this week. Let her hear you tell someone else how lucky you are to have this woman in your life. She may act embarrassed at the time, but she'll love you for it.
3. Prove your love with something tangible. Go out of your way. Sacrifice time, effort, or money to show her how special and unique she is.
4. If she asks for a favor, do it without any objections.
5. Compliment her at least twice this week on her physical beauty. Find something about her appearance that you find attractive and let her know. Remember to be descriptive and specific.
6. Compliment her at least twice this week on what she's done. Pay close attention to all the things she does for you, and take time to recognize them verbally.
7. Pamper her at that special time of the month.
8. Make at least one "I love you" call each day.

Dear Ellen,

Your class on communication saved our marriage. I think it was somewhere around the birth of our second child (we have four) that Justin became completely dedicated to gaining financial security for our family. At the same time, I was knee-deep in diapers, toys, and casseroles. We completely lost touch with one another. The days turned into weeks, then months, and finally years of two strangers living in the same house.

After taking your class, Justin suggested that we go for a walk together each night and see if we couldn't get to know each other again. Ellen, I fell in love with my husband all over again. I had forgotten what a kind, gentle, loving man he really was, and he had forgotten how funny and witty I could be. I feel like the luckiest woman alive to have been given a second chance at loving the same man I've lived with for twelve years.

Love,
Loretta

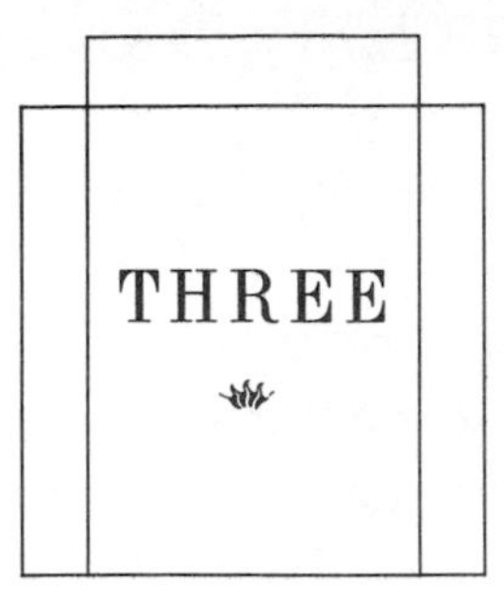

# THREE

## *Listen With All Your Heart*

### SOMEONE TALKS, SOMEONE LISTENS

In nine years of teaching classes for men and women, I can't remember even one man complaining that his wife didn't talk to him enough. In fact, I hear just the opposite. "She never stops talking."

My husband can summarize a two-hour movie in one minute. On the other hand, I would need at least an hour to give you a proper review. To this day, he can't understand how I can go to lunch with a girlfriend and spend three hours talking. Many times he has said, "I don't understand what you can possibly talk about for three hours when you just saw her this past weekend."

As my women's class sessions close, I often warn the women that when their mate asks how the class went, he's not looking for a detailed, blow-by-blow description. All he really wants is a few short sentences telling him what happened. Women have the tendency, because of their enthusiasm, to go home, sit him down, and give him a word-by-word explanation of every minute. This tendency, this need to explain more than you might think necessary, is basic to virtually all women.

I have a much greater need to talk than my husband does. I will talk anywhere to anyone. I am not selective at all. By the time I get off a plane, I've become good friends with the passenger next to me. I talk to people in movie theater lines, the doctor's waiting room, supermarkets, and parking lots. I figure there are millions of stories out there, and I want to get to know as many of them as possible.

My husband is very selective about who he talks to and doesn't have the slightest curiosity about a stranger's life. As far as he's concerned, our telephone is there for business calls and emergencies. He can make appointments with it or arrange an evening with friends, and it's good to have if the family needs to reach us, but it does not provide him with the hours of entertainment my daughters and I seem to derive from it.

Let me remind you again that opposites usually attract. There is no problem being with someone whose style complements yours. Can you imagine how bored to death two people would be if neither talked? But if both were talkers, they'd continually compete with one another to get a word in edgewise.

Any problem you might have with communication in your relationship is not necessarily caused by your differences, but by a lack of understanding or appreciation of those differences. Your ability to verbalize or not has nothing to do with the intensity of your feelings. If someone is more comfortable listening, it doesn't mean he or she feels any less intense than the partner who talks. Don't confuse words, or the lack of them, with emotions. Just because someone doesn't talk much doesn't mean that person's not interested.

In the beginning of your relationship, your different styles didn't concern you. One of you may be a very private person who doesn't feel that his life is anyone else's business. The other may feel compelled to open up to anyone he meets. One of you may talk first and think later. The other may choose his words carefully and wouldn't dream of talking before going over it in his own mind first. One of you may speak very loudly and forcefully. The other may tend to speak softly. Think of your differences as complements, just as you did in the beginning, and you'll be on the right track.

## COURTSHIP CONVERSATION

When a couple first begins dating, there is usually no problem with conversation. In fact, one of the things I always ask a couple is, "Tell me how you met." They describe their first date, and invariably one will say, "And we stayed up half the night just talking" or "We were supposed to go somewhere after dinner, but we just stayed and talked until the restaurant closed."

In the beginning, a couple pays no attention to who began the conversation or who had more to talk about. What they do notice is how comfortable they are with each other, how safe they feel telling each other things they had never shared with anyone else, and how they feel they have known each other all their lives. Their dates are followed by phone calls that sometimes last hours.

Megan described her first date with Mark. "We met at a friend's party. He asked me to dance and then got me a drink. We sat down on the couch and began talking. The next thing I knew, everyone else was leaving. I couldn't believe we spent about three hours talking and laughing. He was so easy to talk to. I found him to be so interesting, and he seemed to like what I had to say. We were so tuned in to each other. He called the next night, and we spent two hours on the phone."

A couple usually falls in love as a result of quality time spent alone talking to each other. They eagerly share their opinions, interests, backgrounds, careers, likes, dislikes, goals, dreams, hopes, fears, and disappointments. Neither judges the other at this point. They're just trying to find out all they can about each other. In this wonderful process of sharing who they are and revealing themselves openly, they both begin to feel very special, loved, and accepted.

You don't have to be a psychologist to be able to look around in any restaurant and guess which couples have been together only a short time and which ones have spent many years together. I'm a people watcher, and I love observing human behavior. As many times as I've seen it, I'm still amazed at a couple who have dinner at a good restaurant and don't say one word to each other the entire evening.

## WHY DID IT STOP?

Couples don't take a vow of silence when they get married. In fact, many men and women look at their parents, who have stopped talking to each other, and say to themselves, "I'm never going to be like them."

So, what happened? How did these couples get to be like their parents, never talking to each other?

Women seem to enjoy conversation for its own sake. It's an end in itself. There are no ulterior motives. Many times I've set up a business luncheon with another woman, we discuss our business, and then we enjoy another hour of what a man would describe as "idle chatter." I learn about her life and problems, and she gets to know mine. By the time we leave, we both share feelings of warmth and understanding. I've made many new friends throughout my life this way.

Most men, on the other hand, seem to engage in conversation as a means to an end. While dating, a man usually has no problem talking, because he has a goal in mind. He wants her to find him desirable, so he's charming, witty, and pays a great deal of attention to what she's saying. He wants to discover what her needs are so that he can fulfill them. As a result, he has a woman who finds him irresistible. Once this happens and she's his forever, he stops talking. In his mind, there's less need to talk and listen to her than there was in the beginning.

Shelley expressed the same concern I've heard from many other women. She said, "I can't understand why Spence, who is a salesman by profession, finds it easy to talk all day long to his customers and can't find anything to talk about when he comes home." For Spence, and countless other men, conversation stops when he's finished his job at the end of the day.

One evening in class, Walter described his feelings, and I think this represents how many men feel. "All day long I try to earn a living. I discuss, I evaluate, I critique, I talk.

I really don't feel like coming home to more of the same. All I want is some peace and quiet. I really think I deserve that."

It is not enough for a woman to have a man who says, "I'm home, aren't I? What more do you want?" If you think that your gift to a woman is giving her the chance to watch you eat, sleep, and sit in front of the TV, you're in for a big surprise.

Speaking of television, a few years ago a report stated that the average American family has the TV on almost seven hours a day, or forty-nine hours a week. The same report said that the average American couple talks only about twenty minutes a week, including the "good mornings," "good nights," and "what do you want for dinners." That's approximately three minutes a day.

One evening, Nancy contributed a humorous example that is all too typical. She provided the women with a reenactment of her husband's homecoming every evening and added her own thoughts between the lines of conversation.

" 'Hi, I'm home,' says Byron. I think, Big deal!" Nancy began.

"Then he always asks, 'How was your day?' and I say okay. I really want to tell him it was great, because I had this hot, torrid love affair today with the mailman.

"He says, 'What's for dinner?' and I tell him chicken, fish, or whatever. I want to say, 'I don't know. What are you cooking tonight?'

"Then he says, 'Any mail?' and I tell him it's on the counter. I want to tell him I got a love letter from the mailman. You should hear what he wants to do to me tomorrow!"

She was quite an amusing actress, but I sensed that all the

women there seemed to identify with what she was saying.

Nancy had every right to expect that Bryon, who had been a clever, witty conversationalist when they first met, would remain so for the rest of their lives together. A relationship that consists of three minutes of conversation a day is headed for disaster. Think about it. Could your job survive on three minutes of work each day? If you wanted to learn new skills, could you learn anything at all if you devoted only three minutes a day to practicing them?

If I want to know how good a couple's sex life is, all I have to ask is, "How good is your conversation together?" A man who takes time to talk to his mate has a responsive woman. If you want a woman who is passionate in the bedroom, you have to learn to fulfill her needs outside the bedroom on a daily basis.

## THIRTY MINUTES A DAY

You may want to relax and unwind by yourself when you come home from work, and you deserve that time alone. If you are living with a woman, you have to take her needs into consideration. She needs to have quality time alone with you every day. I didn't say once in a while. I said *every day.* In fact, there has to be a minimum of thirty minutes each day when she can talk to you and share her experiences and concerns with you. This thirty minutes a day cannot be a monologue. It has to be a dialogue between the two of you. You cannot be just an observer; you have to participate in the conversation too. You need to share some of your own experiences and concerns with her.

When I make this statement in the men's class, I always

notice the reactions of the men who are in a new relationship or about to be married versus the men who have been married for many years. The men in the first group don't even flinch, while the other group moans, groans, and sighs.

One night Neal muttered something to himself. When I asked what it was, he said, "How could you not want to spend at least thirty minutes with the woman you love? I can't wait to see Cathy after work."

In contrast, Roger, a veteran of an eighteen-year marriage, cringed as he said, "You've got to be kidding. If I gave her thirty minutes, she'd want three hours. You don't know my wife."

I may not know his wife, but I did know she was involved in every committee she could find and spent hour after hour talking on the phone. I know that about her because in previous classes Roger had complained about his wife's monopolizing the phone. Her need to talk was being met, just not by her own husband.

## A WOMAN IS LIKE A GARDEN

Jonathan was a delightful man in his seventies and had met his present bride at a social event in the retirement community where he lived. In a beautiful account of how to care for someone, he shared his thoughts. "I lost what I thought was going to be my lifelong mate many years ago. There's no way to explain the alienation and loneliness I felt. When there's no one who cares what kind of a day you had or how bad you're feeling or what you're thinking, it's hard to find a reason to go on living, but you do. Just last year I met Eva, and for you youngsters here, I'm going to tell you that you should never take your wife for granted, no matter how old you are. I count every minute we can be together as very precious. A woman is like a garden. If you don't cultivate her, all you'll get is weeds!"

A man who learns to take time out every day to talk to the woman he loves will win her heart forever. The man who chooses to ignore her need for conversation will find an angry, fault-finding mate. When she nags at you and won't give you a moment's peace, what she's really saying is, "If I can't matter to you with a pleasant conversation, I'll matter through an unpleasant conversation. I'll matter either through communication or conflict, because even conflict is better than the nothingness I feel when I'm around you."

Susan admitted, "I've become a witch. I don't know why Ernest even bothers to come home. All I do is find fault and nag him to death. I guess, in some weird way, I'm still connecting with him, even though we're yelling. I don't think we'd utter any sounds at all if it weren't for our screaming at one another."

Since you're going to spend at least thirty minutes at home anyway, why not choose to have a positive experience instead of a negative one?

If you have children, dinner usually means family conversation and focuses on what the kids have done. This kind of conversation is different from the thirty minutes you need to spend with her. You must take the time for the two of you to be alone.

- If you have to, hire a baby-sitter so the two of you can go out for a walk. There's nothing like a hand-in-hand walk to promote relaxation and conversation. It's also good exercise.

- Take a drive in the car, and pull over to some secluded spot.
- Take her to an informal restaurant for a cup of coffee.
- Sit down in your favorite room, turn off the TV, put on some soft music, and just talk.

Remember, *talk at least thirty minutes each day—no excuses are acceptable.* If you have to go away on a business trip, you can substitute a thirty-minute phone call. Just make sure it's at a time when you know she can be alone with you. If you have children, you'll have to make two phone calls, one to the kids from their dad, but the other is to a woman from her lover.

Sean went home from class feeling very skeptical about the thirty minutes he was going to devote to his wife, but he came back the next week with a smile. "I can't believe what a difference my commitment made. At first, I was doing it for my wife's sake, but soon I found that I was also benefiting from our exclusive time together. Dorine and I decided to take a walk after dinner. We put our fifteen-year-old daughter in charge of our two younger children, and out the door we went. As I began to talk about my concerns and the conflict at work, I was amazed to find out how attentive and supportive Dorine was. This made me feel warm and close to her for the first time in many years. I actually found myself wanting to know more about her day as well. An unexpected result of our nightly walks was a reduction in my irritability and tension. I found myself looking forward to our time together."

Roland, who travels a great deal for his company, made a point of calling his wife late at night after the children were asleep. He took a few moments prior to his phone call to think about how much he missed his wife and what she meant to him. When he called, he was very loving and got a wonderful response. As a result of their intimate conversation and the promise they made to each other that they would connect every day he was away, he said, "I really looked forward to my coming home that week."

For Brent, the thirty minutes a day represented an opportunity to get back in touch with the personal side of his relationship. Both Jana and he were striving to get up the corporate ladder in their respective careers. They had lost all sense of intimacy. Their decision to take a nightly break at a nearby coffee shop was just the remedy they needed to recapture the romance they once had. "Our lovemaking," he confided, "which was infrequent and routine, has become spontaneous and exciting once again, now that we have rediscovered each other."

We're all familiar with the well-worn but true phrase, "It's not the quantity of time you spend, it's the quality of time you spend that counts." Stop and think about it. Are you spending quality time? Sean, Roland, and Brent have all found that one of the secrets to turning a woman on, to bringing out all the softness and responsiveness that she is capable of, is to devote thirty minutes out of each twenty-four hours exclusively to her. Try it and enjoy the rewards that await you.

## YOUR SHOULDER, NOT YOUR MOUTH

I saw a cartoon many years ago that showed a husband reading the newspaper with a frown on his face, and his wife was standing impatiently in front of him. The caption underneath read, "Do we have to save our marriage while I'm reading the sports page?"

Frequently your mate will come to you with what she thinks is a catastrophe or a dilemma, and yes, she may be overreacting or be too emotional, but it's important that you stop what you're doing and pay attention to her. I can promise you that if you stop and take five minutes to hear her out, validate what she's feeling, and comfort her, you'll have at least five hours of peace and quiet. On the other hand, if you're too busy or too tired, you'll probably have five hours of nonstop complaining and arguing.

The formula looks like this,

*Five minutes of my time = Five hours of peace*

Not a bad equation.

Russ agreed with the equation and said, "It was five after eleven, and I was just about to drift off to sleep when I felt my wife gently tapping my shoulder, asking me if I was awake. I pretended I was already asleep. Again, a nudge at my shoulder asking if I was asleep. I just grunted, hoping, once again, that the voice calling me would stop. It didn't. Janice gave me one more tap and said, 'I really need to ask you something. Please get up.' I turned over and tried to focus my eyes on her. She proceeded to tell me how worried she was about the dinner she had to give for my sales group and their wives the following Saturday. 'I've decided on the menu, but I just don't know whether I should serve it buffet style and let everyone get their own food or have a sit-down dinner and serve them.' Wanting to get this over with, I simply said it didn't matter and rolled over. What a mistake!

"Looking back on it now, I wish I had known then what Ellen has taught me, because I would have gotten a good night's rest. As it turned out, this simple question led to an argument that finally ended at three A.M., with both of us emotionally exhausted. She accused me of not caring about anyone but myself and using her as nothing more than a servant. She started crying and screaming that she had had it. Here she was, trying to do something extra special for me, and all I could do was worry about my precious sleep. Well, she was going to see to it that since she was up worrying, I would be also. All night long the accusations went on, I attacking her and her insecurities, she attacking me for my insensitivity. Finally drained, both of us just fell asleep."

All day long you are paid for coming up with solutions, giving advice, and solving problems. When it comes to your personal life, you have to learn to do something completely different. Whenever your mate comes to you with worry, hurt, pain, disappointment, embarrassment, or a problem, she wants you to validate her feelings. What she's saying every time is this: "Listen to me, please. I want to share what happened to me or what I'm worried about. I don't really want any advice or solutions. I just want you to listen to me and understand what I'm saying and care about how I'm feeling."

Memorize this point, and you'll enjoy knowing how easy it is to avoid many of the arguments that now take place in your relationship. Ninety-five percent of the time, your mate isn't looking for answers, she's looking for compassion and sympathy. *She needs your shoulder to lean on, not your mouth to provide answers.*

Once my graduates have learned this, they can't believe what a relief it is not to have to be brilliant. Save your brilliance for your job. It's not necessary in your home.

Stewart came to class very proud of himself after making use of his new knowledge. Every year, his mother came for a two-week stay at his house. She was a widow, and he felt sorry for her and didn't think it was any big deal for his wife, Elsie, to go out of her way for such a short time. Every year, Elsie would complain about what an intrusion on her time and privacy his mother was. And every year Stewart and Elsie fought for a week prior to his mother's arrival and for a week after her departure.

This year was different, because Stewart had just learned to give Elsie his shoulder, not his mouth. When he came home from work, Elsie started her ritual of complaining, but instead of his annual accusation that she was selfish and uncaring, Stewart decided to use what he had learned in class. When Elsie started in, saying, "In one week she'll be here, and look at this place—it's a mess! You know what a stickler your mother is for neatness," Stewart put his arms around her and said, "I know. She's so hard to please. It puts such a strain on you every year. She's so critical and demanding. I know how much you dread her visits. I'm so sorry you always have to go through this."

To his amazement, Elsie melted in his arms, and he couldn't believe his ears when she replied, "It won't be so bad. After all, she is your mother, and without her, you wouldn't have been born, and I'm thankful for that."

Craig is a fisherman one week out of the year. He can't wait to join his three buddies and go on their yearly visit to a nearby stream. "What a hard time Diane gives me every year prior to my going. My reaction up to now has been, 'Please don't start. Whether you like it or not, I'm going. If you don't like it, lump it.' " Craig softened up quite a bit as he, too, applied this new technique.

He can always tell when Diane is about to explode. She starts slamming the cabinets and huffs and puffs around the house. This time, instead of waiting for the barrage of verbal abuse, he went up to her in the kitchen while she was doing the dishes, slipped his arms around her waist, gave her a kiss, and said, "Sweetheart, I know it's very selfish of me to go fishing. I leave you with all the chores and responsibilities while I go and have fun. It's really not fair. You really mean the whole world to me, and if it upsets you this much, I'll cancel my trip. It's really not worth it. You are the most important person in my life and mean more than a fishing trip."

How could this woman not be moved by such a compassionate, understanding man? There was no doubt in my mind what Diane would say, but Craig was shocked later that evening when she finally responded to his words.

As they got ready for bed, Diane said, "Well, I've been thinking. I really do want you to go, because it seems to relax you so much. I just want you to understand that it's a burden on me, and besides, I miss you so much."

Craig agreed to take Diane away for the weekend after he got back so that he could make it up to her.

## THE ART OF LISTENING

When you really learn the art of listening, when you learn to suspend your own thoughts and feelings in order to hear what your mate is saying, you begin to see things from another point of view. A relationship is composed of two different people who have to make a decision to try to see things through their mate's eyes. If you try to put yourself in her place, to see things the way she sees them for just a moment, your reaction to what she says or does will be very different. Good listening promotes closeness and understanding. When she knows you understand how she feels, not just what she's saying, when she talks to you and you let her know it's okay to have those feelings, that woman feels so satisfied. In return, she will want to do anything in her power to make you happy.

## THE PAST IS OVER

If you have been lucky enough to have a woman who felt it was safe to share her past with you because she trusted you, don't make her sorry she did. If you do, she'll never open herself up again. Sometimes women will take a leap of faith and be completely honest with you about their past. If you are not understanding and sympathetic, it will be the last time they take that chance.

Darin admitted how insensitive he had been. "When I asked Darlene how many men she had slept with before she met me, she told me there had been three. I just about hit the roof. She tried to explain that she had been young and naïve, but I wouldn't listen. I refused to believe her when she told me that no man had ever made her feel as complete as I did. I got madder and madder the more I thought about it. Every time we made love, I felt like I was in competition with her past lovers, and sometimes I would even ask her how I compared with them. I now know how sorry she must have been that she had told me the truth. I only hope I can reassure her that I know I was wrong to react like that. I'm never going to bring it up again."

Cindy revealed how sorry she was for telling Joel that she used to be very heavy as a teen-ager, that it wasn't until her late twenties that she gained control of her problem. "Now he watches me like a hawk. Every time I have dessert, he'll bring up my past and throw it in my face. Boy, was I stupid to confide in him."

For Melvin, this lesson came at the perfect time. He and his girlfriend, Amanda, had been dating for two years. He had asked her to marry him a month prior to his taking the class, but she had put him off. She needed more time. One evening after he had started my classes, she called and said she needed to talk, could he come over right away. She confessed that she had been hiding something from him since the day they met. "Amanda told me she never finished high school," he said. "I honestly think I might have gotten upset if I hadn't taken your class. After all, we had discussed our high school experiences many times, and I had just assumed that she had graduated. Instead, I took her in my arms and told her how glad I was that she felt safe enough to confide in me and that I loved her even more for trusting me enough to do that. For the next four hours, she told me about the agony of her home life as a teen-ager, how it was so bad that she could never concentrate in class. It finally became too much, and she got a job as a receptionist. She has moved up in the company and is now a supervisor.'' The wonderful part of this story is that soon after Amanda opened up, she and Melvin set a date for their wedding.

The past is over, and it can't be changed. We all come into relationships with excess baggage, things we'd like to change and experiences we wish we'd never had. Your tenderness and love has the ability to heal her wounds and to make her feel whole again. Don't waste that precious ability. It's a gift you can give her for the rest of your life together.

## DON'T SHOULD ON ME

I once saw a wonderful bumper sticker that said, ''Don't Should On Me.''

There's nothing more upsetting for a woman than coming to the one person she loves more than anyone else in this whole world, telling you about an incident that just happened, and having you react by saying, ''You should have done this instead.''

Linda explained that her boss was too critical and demanding, and one day she just couldn't stand it anymore and quit. ''When I came home and explained what had happened, Ben told me I shouldn't have quit without looking for another job first. He didn't see that my immediate reaction was not clear, logical thinking, but an emotional response to a bad situation. I thought he'd be understanding, but instead I felt like all I did was disappoint him. I wish that he had just held me and told me that he loved me.''

Here are a few more examples that have come from the classroom.

*She says:* "What a lousy day I had at work."

*Wrong response:* "Well, you should just quit that dumb job. It's not like we need the money."

*Right response:* "My poor sweetheart. Tell me what happened. They just don't appreciate what a wonderful employee they have in you."

*She says:* "What a miserable day I had with the kids. Johnny was throwing up all day, and I finally took him to the doctor. Penny didn't help matters. All she did was act like a spoiled brat because I wasn't paying her any attention. I'm so tired."

*Wrong response:* "You should be thankful you don't have to go to work all day like I do. You think you have it rough, wait until I tell you about my day."

*Right response:* "Sweetheart, you must be exhausted. Trying to cope with one child who's sick and another who demands your attention must be so frustrating. I don't know how you do it. I'm so lucky to have such a wonderful wife, and those kids are darn lucky to have one terrific mother."

*She says:* "I'm so nervous about going to the doctor. I'm scared he'll find something wrong with me."

*Wrong response:* "There's nothing to worry about. You should just tell yourself that everything will be okay. You know that negative thinking does you no good."

*Right response:* "Oh, baby, I know how upset you are. You're filled with anxiety and worry. Come here and let me hold you in my arms."

In the above examples, the wrong responses all disregard the woman's feelings. When you "should" on her, the messages she gets from you are:

- You don't think my feelings are important.
- You think my feelings are wrong.
- You don't understand my feelings at all.

The effects of this type of communication on your part will be anger and resentment on her part. On the other hand, if you learn how to respond to her feelings the right way, the messages you send to her are:

- You have every right to express how you feel.
- I respect your feelings.
- I really see your point of view.
- I understand and care about your feelings.

The effects of this type of communication on your part will be love and appreciation on her part.

In times of stress, your arms do more to comfort her than any other part of your body. She needs to be held, not given a lecture. A good way to remember this is a quote I once heard: "God gave us two ears and one mouth, which means we must learn to listen twice as much as we talk." Another wonderful way of thinking about communication is that our mouths open and close, but our ears are designed to just stay open. So listen to her. It will be good for both of you.

Sometimes your mate will want you to help her solve a problem or give her the solution to a dilemma. The message will be very clear. It will be something like, "Hon, please tell me what to do in this case." Or perhaps she will say, "Sweetheart, I really need your help in solving this problem." This will be true only about 5 percent of the time. The other 95 percent of the time, she just wants you to show that you care, that you understand what she's saying and want to validate her feelings.

## NONVERBAL CLUES

Years ago, Eastman Kodak Company did a study to find out what we do when we try to communicate. They found out that:

- Words make up only 7 percent of the message we're trying to give.
- Nonverbal communication, which consists of smiles, stares, glares, and frowns, was 55 percent of the total message.
- Tone of voice was the other 38 percent of the message.

Children are really good at picking up nonverbal clues, which are the biggest indicators of what you are communicating. Patrick said that his four-year-old daughter came over to him, sat on his lap, and asked him what was wrong. When he replied nothing, she put both hands on his cheeks and said, "Then why don't you tell your face that?"

Paying attention to nonverbal clues usually gives you more insight into what your mate is feeling and will actually give you a more accurate message than the words coming out of her mouth. Every man faced with a woman who is slamming doors or throwing dishes can guess that his mate is angry, but it takes a little more effort to notice more subtle clues, such as rigid movements in her walk, no expression on her face, staring out into space, rolling her eyes, or shrugging her shoulders in response to a statement. If a woman avoids your eyes, you can be sure something is bothering her. If she distances herself physically from you or makes no attempt to touch you, it's another sure bet she's upset at something.

Here again, the five-minute principle will be worth your time and effort. The equation this time is:

*Five minutes of my time = Five hours of harmony*

If you suspect that something is wrong, try to nip it in the bud. Don't ignore it, because it will only build up to a greater intensity. This one is really a challenge and probably will exhaust you, but don't give up. I promise it won't take more than five minutes. When you first ask her what is wrong, her answer will be "nothing." Her tone of voice will be a dead giveaway if you are a perceptive man.

Ask the question again, only this time add, "Please tell me what's wrong. I know something is bothering you."

Once again, her answer will be, "I told you; nothing is wrong."

Don't get discouraged. It's almost like a test she has to put you through. Your persistence means you care about her, and she secretly loves the fact that you are spending extra time and effort on her.

This time, add, "Please tell me what's wrong. I must have done something to hurt you, and unless I know what it is, I can't do anything about it."

She's weakening at this point, I promise. Now, in your final attempt, say, "Please, please tell me what's wrong so I can make it up to you. You're the most important person in my life, and I love you with all my heart. Sometimes I can be insensitive to you, and I just need to know what happened."

The hardest part about this is that right now you may have spent only three minutes pleading, and you have two more to go, but keep trying. The reward will be worth it. She'll finally let you know, you'll have a chance to discuss it, she'll feel better, and it will be over.

The alternative is so much worse. If you ignore her clues or take her "nothing" literally, you'll live with an angry, cold woman who is capable of distancing herself from you for hours, even days.

Your persistence will pay off. The more you show concern for her by asking her what's wrong, the easier telling you will get for her. Most women will eventually learn to tell you immediately what's bothering them, and the five minutes it used to take will diminish to about two seconds.

## YOU THOUGHT I MEANT IT?

Communication is really an art. Sometimes it requires that you make a distinction between what she says and what she really means. Quite often these two are completely unrelated. From time to time most women are guilty of saying one thing and meaning something else. To make matters worse, they expect you to have ESP and know automatically what they really meant, even if they didn't say it. Since you probably don't have this ability, or at least the majority of men I've met don't have it, a good rule of thumb is just to assume that, most of the time, *what she says is not really what she means.*

For some reason, you are expected to know this. One possible explanation for her expectation is that in a scientific project, the researchers found that most women are more intuitive than men. They catch subliminal messages three times faster than men. Remember your mother knowing something was wrong even when you were trying to hide it from her? As soon as you walked in the door, she could tell something had happened.

It's human nature to assume that everyone else possesses the same abilities we have. Since most women can usually read between the lines or catch a double meaning in what is being said, chances are that the woman in your life expects the same of you.

I've never met a man who didn't eventually develop his perceptive abilities as a result of his mate making his life miserable if he didn't. I, too, was guilty of expecting my husband to be able to read my mind.

When we first got married, money was scarce, and as our first anniversary approached I said, "Let's not get each other anything." He took what I said literally. The special day arrived, and there I was with a card and a gift for him. He, of course, had nothing for me, because that's what I had asked.

I burst into tears, and my poor husband stood there feeling like an idiot, saying, "But you said we shouldn't get each other anything!" My response was, "And you thought I meant it? How could you possibly think that's what I meant? I meant we didn't have to spend a lot of money, but I guess, since I must mean nothing to you, it was easier to just believe me."

Does this sound familiar? If you have a choice between doing something nice for her and doing nothing, giving her a gift or not giving one, always do the nice thing and always go get that gift, no matter what she has said. You can bet that every time she says not to bother getting her a gift, she secretly wants one. Every time she says, "Don't go out of your way for me," that is exactly what you should do.

Mike, my daughter's boyfriend, has learned to read her mind in a very short time. She had come home from college for a long weekend and he flew to California to stay with us for a few days. The evening before she was to return to college, she told him that since he had a later flight than she did, he didn't need to take her to the airport. Her father would do that, and Mike could just sleep late. The next morning, I was surprised to see Mike up early, taking her to the airport. When he got back to the house, I asked why he had decided to do that, since my husband had agreed to take her on his way to work. Mike looked at me with his adorable blue eyes and said, "Are you kidding? If I had slept in, I would never hear the end of it. She would have thought I was selfish and uncaring. I now know that whatever Tara says, I do just the opposite!" This wise young man has learned in only a short time what it has taken some men years to figure out.

The night before, I honestly believed that my daughter didn't care who took her to the airport. Later, in a phone conversation, I asked her whether it had really mattered to her. "Of course it mattered," she said. "I really did want

Mike to take me, and yes, I would have gotten upset if he hadn't!"

Barney, on the other hand, still had a bit to learn. He and his wife went window shopping for her birthday present. When a beautiful watch caught her eye, she dragged him inside to get a closer look. Upon learning the price of the watch, she said, "Oh, that's too expensive," and she began looking at a less expensive watch. When she selected an alternative that was half the price, Barney was ecstatic. Here was a woman after his own heart, concerned about their finances and being very sensible and frugal.

The day of her birthday, he presented her with this bargain and found, to his joy, a wife who began to cry. Thinking these were tears of happiness, he put his arms around her, but to his surprise, she shoved him away. "How could you?" she said. "You knew how much I wanted the other watch, and you went out and bought this one. I would never have done that to you." The ironic part of this story is that he would have gladly bought her initial choice if he had only known. He said, "I honestly thought she didn't want it because it was too expensive. I was trying to please her. Well, I've learned a valuable lesson."

Most stories like this are usually humorous when you hear them, but humor is the last thing that comes to mind when they are actually happening.

Miles said that before Christmas, his wife hinted that she wanted a dog. "But I guess because she knew I didn't care for animals that much, Nadine said that a stuffed animal would do. I spent a great deal of time looking for a cute stuffed dog. When she opened the package on Christmas morning, she began laughing and looking around for the puppy she thought I had hidden. When I assured her that there wasn't one, she looked at me with a shocked expression and said, 'You mean you spent money on this pretend dog when you knew I wanted the real thing? Would you like me to walk it on a leash?' I didn't believe what I was hearing at first, but I finally got the message. The next day, I told her to sit down on the couch, close her eyes, and hold her arms out. When she felt the new addition to our household, she was obviously the happiest woman alive. She didn't stop kissing me all day long."

Here's a quick course in ESP. If you hear the following words, you can assume she means the opposite.

> *She says:* "Oh, honey, you don't have to do that."
> Yes, you do!
> *She says:* "Sweetheart, that's too much money."
> No, it isn't!
> *She says:* "That's okay, it's too much of an inconvenience for you."
> No it isn't!
> *She says:* "No, don't bother."
> Do bother!
> *She says:* "I don't really care."
> She cares!
> *She says:* "Tell me the truth."
> Watch out!

Anything that makes her feel special and worth going to some trouble for is not going to go unrecognized.

She may ask you about her physical appearance and begin with, "Tell me the truth."

> How do I look?
> Do you think I'm getting old?

Do you think I'm getting heavy?
Do you think I'm beginning to sag?

I'm not asking you to lie, but do understand that the real reason she's asking is to get some assurance that you still find her attractive. Diplomacy and your choice of words can go a long way. Of course beauty is in the eye of the beholder, and I would hope your eyes capture something beautiful to behold! Here's where the following statements would be of great value.

- To me, you'll always be my beautiful bride.
- You're not getting older, you're getting better.
- You always turn me on.
- You are the sexiest woman alive.
- I'm lucky to have a wonderful woman like you.
- How did I ever deserve someone as special as you?
- That color brings out those big, beautiful brown (or blue) eyes.

When I left home to get married, I had never cooked a complete meal in my life. My mother always took care of that, and I simply had no desire to learn. After our honeymoon, I prepared my first dinner. I actually bought a cookbook geared to teen-agers, called *Let's Begin to Cook.* I still have it on my shelf as a reminder of how far I've come. I did not know how to boil an egg, cook a roast, or even sauté an onion. I decided to make meatballs and spaghetti, and it took me all day. The recipe called for a clove of garlic, but I didn't know that meant one piece of garlic; I thought it meant the whole bulb. After hours of tender loving care, I finally served this gourmet delight. I took my first bite and almost died. I had used enough garlic to cause bad breath for a year. I knew I had married a special man when he took his first bite and said it was delicious. I couldn't imagine what had gone wrong and wanted to throw the whole meal in the garbage, but he looked me square in the eye and said, "Honey, you went to all this trouble for me, and I want you to know I love you for it."

He continued to eat. Can you imagine how much concentration it took for him to focus on his love and sensitivity to me, rather than on that awful meal?

A word to the wise is sufficient here. Find something about her you love, why she makes a difference in your life, and how she matters more than anyone else, and you'll never deviate from the truth. I wish you happiness as you develop your intuitive ability with her, as you learn to understand what she really means, and in all your future communication.

## ACTION ASSIGNMENT #3

1. Plan to spend a minimum of thirty minutes each day talking with her. Ask her about her day and really listen. Let her know you understand and care. Then it will be your turn to share your day with her.
2. If she comes to you with a problem or complaint, really listen and repeat what she's just said in your own words. Then, put your arms around her and just hold her.
3. Pay attention to nonverbal clues this week to see if your mate is happy or angry. If you think she's angry or upset about something, sit down with her and probe. Don't leave her side until she confesses what's on her mind.

Dear Ellen,

How can it be possible to turn a man who never listened to me, had no compassion, and always thought he was right into an understanding, thoughtful, compassionate husband in just five weeks? Every day, I pinch myself just to see if I'm dreaming. Are you sure you don't use hypnosis in your class?

Love,
Connie

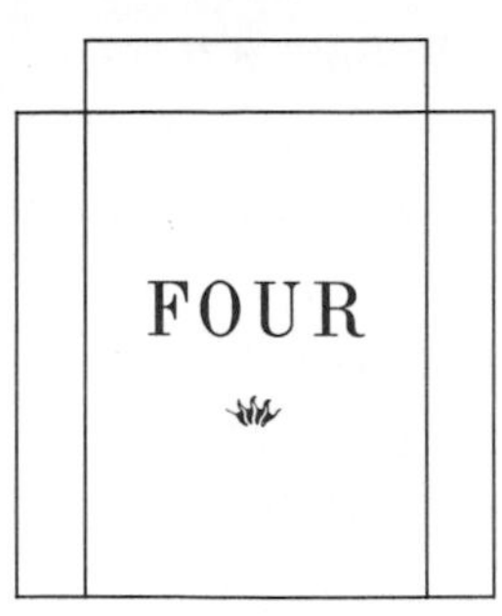

# FOUR

# *Nothing More Than Feelings*

## FEELINGS ARE NOT GOOD BUSINESS

Success at your job probably depends on your ability to suppress your feelings. In most situations at work, you have to be controlled, calculating, deliberate, and sometimes even manipulative. If you showed your real feelings, you'd probably be fired and replaced by someone who was more dehumanized.

Louis came to class one evening looking as if he had just lost his dog. When I questioned him, he sadly confirmed, "Yes, I'm upset about something. I just got fired today. I rent executive office space, and the man who owns the building felt I wasn't forceful enough with prospective tenants. He wanted someone who was able to close the deal immediately, no matter what the cost. He told me he was getting someone who would not let a client leave without signing on the dotted line. Well, I'm not like that. I develop a rapport with people, and if they want to think it over or feel it's not right for them, I don't try to convince them that this is perfect for them. If price is a concern, I respect their wish to shop around. The owner wanted someone who disregards the tenant and can concentrate only on the buck."

In a society that is concerned with the end and not the means, a man who tends to feel for other people, as well as for himself, often has a difficult time producing results. Many men have said that the advice given to them on their first day of work is, "The bottom line here is results! We don't care what you have to do to get it. Wine, dine, and charm the client, whether you like him or not."

Derrick, who chose a career in the military, remembered, "I felt really lousy about being married. I was told that if they had wanted me to have a wife, they would have issued me one! They were saying that they didn't care about our roles as husbands or fathers. All they cared about was us being good soldiers. Our personal lives were of no concern to them, and we had better be able to disassociate ourselves from it if we wanted to stay."

Rhett was a third-year medical student, and his comment was, "Nobody cares that you've been up for two days straight and are at the point of exhaustion. You can't see straight, let alone think about what you're doing. Compassion from others is pretty rare while you're becoming a doctor."

What do you think your chances for a promotion would be if, during the interview, you talked about your fears of not being able to handle the next level, or about your anxiety that another co-worker would get the position instead of you? What man would get the job if he talked about his high blood pressure or about the worries he had at home?

You'd have to present yourself as a capable, knowledgeable, and assertive man in order to win over the competition. Success in your professional life sometimes means being devoid of feelings. But your professional life is not your personal life, and you have to make a distinction between them.

## STICKS AND STONES

Success in your personal life means being able to express your feelings, both the good ones and the bad ones. More than anything else, to feel really alive and human depends on your ability to acknowledge your feelings and be comfortable with them.

This is not easy, because from the time you were a little boy, you were taught to deny your feelings. Parents are the greatest teachers in the denial of feelings department. As a young child, you came to them with your hurts and fears, and although there is no difference between how a little girl and a little boy feel, you were taught to believe that there was supposed to be a difference. As a boy, your parents probably reacted to you in a different way than they would have if you had been a little girl. Girls are generally allowed to cry, but boys are ridiculed if they do.

If someone at school called you a name, and you came home crying, you probably heard a common response: "Sticks and stones will break your bones, but names will never harm you."

That's a lie that you tried desperately to believe. The truth is, name-calling hurts. If you were overweight, being called fatso hurt. If it took you a little longer to understand something, being called stupid hurt. If you wore glasses, being called four-eyes hurt. If you were sensitive, being called a sissy, mama's boy, or crybaby hurt.

So, after feeling hurt and sharing that feeling, what did you get? Certainly not sympathy, understanding, and a validation of your feelings. You got "sticks and stones" repeated in an almost mechanical manner. When this happened, you were even more confused, because it was only natural for you to want to please your parents. So you tried not to feel hurt. You eventually pretended that it was no big deal. Ultimately, you learned to cover up your feelings. After all, if you were going to be a man, you weren't going to cry. If you wanted to be loved by your parents, you had to try hard not to be so sensitive.

These were hard lessons to learn. It took a great deal of repetition to get it right. As you got older, you may have voiced a particular feeling you had. Maybe you were afraid of the dark. But instead of having your feelings validated by having a parent say, "I know. Sometimes it's scary to be in the dark. Your imagination plays tricks on you. Let's check out this room together. You know what? We'll leave the hall light on so it's not so scary," what you probably heard was, "Just go to sleep and stop being a scaredy-cat."

Later, as you entered high school and felt anxiety about a test, chances are that at one time you were completely honest with your emotions and told your parents how nervous you were. What response did you get? "If you study, there's nothing to be nervous about." What you needed to hear was, "It's very natural to be nervous about an exam, especially when it's half your grade." Instead of having your feelings validated, you had them discounted.

As a teen-ager, it is very normal to be concerned about your peers and what they think of you. It's a time when you want to blend in and be accepted. If you wanted to wear certain clothes or a certain hairstyle, you probably heard a lecture on being your own person and that what other people think should make no difference. Well, other people *do* affect you, and instead of understanding that this is a time of insecurity for most boys, your parents were probably baffled and disappointed by your concerns.

The lessons continued coming, even as late as your first step toward adulthood. Maybe when you began your first job, you came home and said that it was no fun. So your parents, instead of relating their similar feelings and remembering back to a time when their expectations were not met either, gave you lecture #73 on "What does fun have to do with work!"

## OVERCOMING WHAT YOU'VE BECOME

It's important to understand that your upbringing has a great deal to do with whether you are a man who now finds it easy or difficult to share his feelings. Taking off the mask that you've been hiding behind for years is a frightening experience. Some of you have pushed down your real feelings for so long that you don't even know how capable you are of feeling deeply.

A man who is not able to share his feelings because of the belief that he has to project what he thinks is a male image at all times, that he has to be a *real* man, distances himself from the woman he loves.

Women respect and admire a man for his strength and want someone they can lean on, but they also love a man who can show his vulnerability by sharing his honest feelings. If you don't learn to share who you really are, you won't experience the benefits of having a woman comfort and nurture you.

## SHARING YOUR FEELINGS

A woman loves the feeling of being needed. When a man tells a woman how important she is in his life and how her support and encouragement give him a reason for living, it's probably one of the most romantic statements he can make.

Fifteen years ago, my husband lost his business and we went through bankruptcy. His ego was shattered as he kept looking for work, but without success. I constantly told him how much I believed in him and what a difference he made in my life, as well as in our children's lives. I did everything I could to cheer him up and lighten his heavy burden. My payoff came when he finally obtained a job after many months of searching. He held me in his arms one night and, with tears in his eyes, told me how lucky he was to have me as his wife and that my belief in him had helped him believe in himself. I'd rate that conversation as one of the highlights of my life.

Calvin, who considered himself a good surgeon, told the class how he'd never forget the first time he had a patient die on the operating table. "I had to appear strong and composed as I told the immediate family of this man's death. I also had other surgery that had to be performed that day, so I couldn't give in to my emotions. They had to be set aside for the sake of the other patients that needed me. When I walked through the door that night, I broke down and burst into tears. My wife came over and just held me in her arms. She kept stroking me and telling me how awful it must have been and how sorry she was that I had to go through this. I can't imagine what it would have been like to come home to an empty place with no one to comfort me. I owe her a lot."

Jarvis, a computer salesman, revealed that two years ago he got a really bad job evaluation. "My boss went through a list of traits necessary for success on the job. He gave me checks in the average and poor columns, along with suggestions for improvements needed if I were to remain employed by the company. I left that day feeling complete despair. At first, I wasn't going to tell my girlfriend, because I didn't need her to think I was a dismal failure. I tried to hide what I was feeling, but later that night I finally confessed what had happened. She didn't say much; she just really listened. The next morning when I got up, I found a piece of paper with a list of traits, like honesty, integrity, sensitivity, sense of humor, etc. She'd made columns—poor, fair, above average, and excellent. She had checked excellent on every trait, and at the bottom of the sheet there was a space for other comments. There, she wrote that because I was the best man in her life, I was to receive a special award that night. I can't begin to explain how good I felt the whole day. That evening, she presented me with a plaque that was engraved, 'To the #1 man in my life,' and then she listed the traits she loved."

Give the woman in your life a chance to be needed. Let her know your hopes, dreams, and accomplishments, but also let her share your fears, disappointments, and pain.

Women have come a long way in emancipating their feelings. Now it's your turn. Thank goodness the movie idols of the past, such as Clark Gable, Burt Lancaster, John Wayne, and Kirk Douglas, who were classified as "real men," have now been replaced by Alan Alda, Jack Lemmon, Ed Asner, Tom Hanks, and Tom Cruise. Real men today can show tears and vulnerability. They are the ones women idolize now. A softer man has emerged. In the film *Rocky,* the boxer played by Sylvester Stallone turns to his wife and says, "Hold me—I'm scared."

A courageous man can admit his true feelings. A weak man always hides behind a mask of independence and indifference, distancing himself from the woman he loves.

## YOUR HEALTH DEPENDS ON IT!

Another good reason why it is important to share your feelings is your health. Studies have shown that men who are prone to ulcers, colitis, high blood pressure, heart attacks, and cancer have a greater inability to express their feelings than healthier men. These illness-prone men are usually referred to as good guys. They are the men who usually portray themselves as carefree and laid-back, and eventually, instead of their worries coming out of their mouths, their worries stay in their bodies and cause disease.

In *Love, Medicine and Miracles,* Bernie Segal says that "lack of emotional outlet is a common theme in cancer patients."

Look at the word disease. It is composed of *dis* and *ease.* When you're not at ease, you tend to get sick. One of the best ways to relieve stress is to talk about what's going on. Learn to open up, to talk about how you really feel. You'll be surprised at what it can do for you physically. You'll have a spring in your step and a great deal more energy as you experience this new freedom that is rightfully yours.

## WHAT ELSE IS THERE?

One night, I asked thirty-five men in my class to talk to each other about anything other than work, sports, or current events. Complete silence followed. Finally, I put a list on the board that consisted of the following words.

| | | | |
|---|---|---|---|
| Dating | Mothers | Pleasure | Marrige |
| Fathers | Neighbors | Fantasies | Children |
| Siblings | Fears | Phobias | Best Friends |
| Worries | Temper | Anger | |

Most of the men in the group were surprised that they could not think of these subjects themselves.

When men get together, the question they most often ask each other is "How's it going?" That usually leads into conversation about their jobs, accomplishments, current world problems, weather, or sports.

When women get together, their conversation begins with "How are you?" That leads into hours of discussing their relationships, along with their feelings.

It takes too much energy to spend your whole life covering up feelings to prove that you are independent, assertive, controlled, courageous, competitive, fearless, and carefree at all times. It takes much less energy to reveal who you really are and, in turn, have someone love you for your strengths as well as your vulnerabilities.

If you have a woman who continually tries to find out how you feel, you should realize that she came into your life to help you live a richer, more rewarding, and more fulfilling life. Don't shut her out. This is an area where a woman usually excels and can help you discover the real you. Save your pretend self for your job and strangers. Give your real self to the woman who loves you with all her heart.

Some of the top-rated TV shows are *The Bill Cosby Show, Roseanne, The Wonder Years, Who's the Boss?,* and a new entry, *Married . . . With Children.* Through humor, these shows demonstrate the daily frustrations, anxieties, worries, and joys involved in raising a family and being in a relationship. When Barbara Walters hosts one of her specials, it is the number one choice of millions of viewers. The competition doesn't even come close. Why? Because when Barbara gets through interviewing a celebrity, you feel as if you've learned something about the real person behind the characters he or she portrays. You find out his hopes, dreams, fears, anxieties, failures, and expectations. I don't think she'd attract the viewers she does if she interviewed celebrities to get a detailed account of their day, along with their job description.

Today, the public is devouring memoirs of people in the public eye or biographies about them. *Roseanne* by Roseanne Barr and *It's My Turn* by Nancy Reagan have become immediate best-sellers because people enjoy getting information about what the real person behind the public image is like. Every couple of years a new biography of Jacqueline Onassis comes out and tops the best-seller lists. Never mind that she's never written or authorized any of these. We'll happily accept secondhand accounts as long as we get some new insight into this fascinating woman.

Sometimes, by reading about or listening to someone famous share his disappointments, failures, inadequacies, and mistakes, we are able to tap into our own feelings. The similarities we hear, in a sense, validate our own feelings. We are reassured that what we are feeling is no different from what that successful person is feeling.

The public is fascinated by the real people who lie beneath the roles the stars play, just as your mate is fascinated by the real you. You may not be in the public eye, but you are number one in your sweetheart's life, and she wants to know you inside and out. You may never get to write your memoirs, but you can verbalize them with your mate. The duality of the roles you play is more important to your mate than any actor's role.

Famous people who are strong enough to reveal their weaknesses or share the challenges they've faced in their lives capture the hearts of Americans everywhere. Oprah Winfrey has gained more popularity by sharing her constant struggle to maintain her weight with the public. Betty Ford was an inspiration to many when she explained, firsthand, the problems of alcohol and drug abuse. Tom Cruise has admitted having dyslexia. These people in the public eye are admired for the strength it takes to talk openly about their problems. Why not capture the heart of your woman? Share your hopes and fears and failures with her. Be strong enough to risk exposing who you really are.

## YOUR UNIT OF WORTH

Some men are unable to separate who they are from what they do. During the Great Depression, men committed suicide because they had lost the ability to earn a living and equated that with no longer having a reason to live.

Merle, a youthful man in his late sixties, admitted to being one of those men who contemplated ending his life during that difficult time in our country. He made a lasting impression on me and all his classmates when he made this statement: "Look, with all this women's liberation talk that we've heard in the last two decades, it's still true today that if an elderly couple is penniless and forced to live on welfare and social security checks, no one is going to point the finger at the wife and ask why she didn't provide for the two of them. They'll point the finger at the husband and wonder why he didn't work hard enough so they could enjoy their remaining years. The blame is still on the male!"

Most men in my classes still see themselves as the breadwinner, the one responsible for supporting the family. They still feel that it's up to them to take care of earning a living. If their wives work, they prefer to look at it as a choice, not a necessity. Even when I questioned men who have mates who earn equal salaries or even more than they do, some of the responses have been:

- She can still quit anytime she wants, but I can't.
- She works so we can have the extras in life we couldn't afford if we had only my salary.
- She works so she can feel good about herself. She feels she's useful and contributing.
- It's just a hobby that she's turned into a business.

Most men still believe that they shoulder the major responsibility in providing a stable income. In our society, where the emphasis is on earning more so one can accumulate a bigger pile of material things, is it any wonder that men struggle to get ahead in order to have more value in the eyes of others? Because of this emphasis on achieving wealth, their self-worth is somehow related to their ability to provide a living. If you are to become a truly liberated man, you'll have to replace these old messages with a new one that says, "The work I do is not related to my worth as a human being."

Maybe it will help to look at it this way. Every human being, at the instant he or she is born, is assigned one unit of worth. This one unit does not change when you are sick, out of work, or old. Until the day you take your last breath, you still have that unit of worth. What you do or don't do cannot erase your unit of worth. It's permanent. Does Mother Teresa have less worth because she gets no salary for helping the less fortunate? Does a priest have less value for giving up all his worldly possessions to serve God? Does a child who dies very young have no worth because he was here for only a short time? Does a man like Donald Trump have more worth than a Vietnam War veteran? Is someone who has spent his time building an empire a better man than one who risked his life fighting for his country? The answer is no. We all have a unit of worth.

Many men don't realize that there is just as much worth in raising a child who is a good-natured and respectable member of society as there is in raising their own income. Many men don't realize that bringing happiness to their mate and raising her self-esteem is just as valuable as raising their own position in a company.

There are so many aspects of your life that can give you a sense of value. Being someone's child, grandchild, lover, boyfriend, husband, or father can bring you more joy, sense of accomplishment, and rewards than any job possibly could if you only allow it to happen. No man on his deathbed says, "I should have spent more time at the office. I should have worked harder and done more overtime."

I always get at least a chuckle, if not laughter, when I make that statement, because it is true. Men on their deathbeds talk about what is really important. What is said is, "I should have spent more time and energy on those I loved and those who loved me."

## YOU ARE NOT WHAT YOU DO

A man who feels there is a great disparity between what he does for a living and who he really is tends to be mentally healthier than those who can't seem to separate the two.

Peter Sellers was an acting genius described by friends as a man who never really knew who he was going to be at any given moment. He was always "on," assuming so many different characters that no one could ever be certain what was real and what was just acting.

Robin Williams is another genius and is very difficult to deal with in a conventional way. Even Barbara Walters couldn't get to him. Every time she asked a serious question, he'd change his voice and become someone else, answering in an endearing but joking way. He was also interviewed in *People* magazine, and he said that his young son keeps him grounded. When he starts playing all those different roles, his son will say, "No, I want my daddy, my *real* daddy."

George Burns, on the other hand, has no pretenses. You sense that what you see is what you get. He always talks and writes openly about himself.

It's true that our society demands that we play certain roles. Can you imagine a political candidate running for office admitting that he wanted the position because he loved power, control, money, and fame? What if he voiced certain personal preferences or prejudices? He'd never be elected. Jimmy Carter was blasted by the press because he admitted that there was lust in his heart. Society prefers to think that their president is somehow above such base feelings.

Through the years, many men in my classes have openly discussed the difference between the roles they play at work and their honest, true feelings when they find out it's really okay to have conflicting emotions.

Larry, a plastic surgeon for more than nineteen years, said, "I still feel that when I perform reconstructive surgery on a patient who is born with a defect or has had a terrible accident, I'm really contributing something meaningful. But when a woman comes in my office complaining about the bags under her eyes or the fact that she's getting older and doesn't like it, I really don't have any compassion. I pretend I do, of course, because that's ninety percent of my practice now. I really want to say, 'That's tough. We all get old, lady, including me.' When she wants her breasts enlarged or her tummy tucked, I'd like to show her pictures of people with real problems. But then I'd have no patients, would I? So I pretend to be interested, understanding, and concerned."

Jon, a young man in his early twenties, works for a telemarketing firm. "I've been taught never to be rude to a potential customer, no matter what. Well, you can't believe how rude people are on the telephone. They hang up in the middle of what I'm saying, and I really want to call them back and say, 'Screw you, too!' They let me go through my whole speech and, at the end, tell me they have absolutely no intention of buying anything and how dare I call them. That's when I really get frustrated and want to scream, 'You dummy! Why did you act so interested?' But I don't. I just thank them for taking the time to listen to me."

Vinnie, a car salesman for the past ten years, said, "It's so frustrating to see a man pick out a car he likes and then bring the 'little woman' to see it. She proceeds to tell him how she really doesn't like it, and I politely show them fifty more models. What I really feel is anger and annoyance and a desire to tell this guy he has no balls! Can't he make a decision without her? I'd like to smack her, too, while I'm at it. Of course, I don't. I act like I'm their best friend and only want to see them happy with the choice they make."

Curtis, a psychiatrist with a booming practice in a very wealthy area in California, admitted, "When these rich women come into my office trying to 'find themselves,' it quite often makes me sick. They have nothing but time on their hands and no one to think about but themselves. Sometimes I want to condense their years of analysis into a few minutes where I would tell them to just stop feeling sorry for themselves, to stop thinking about themselves, and to think about how they can help someone else who's really having problems. Obviously, I don't do that, but I sure feel like it."

Barry, a high school football coach who is respected for his talent in turning out a great team every year, said, "I'm so tired and bored. I keep thinking, This is my ninth year, and if I have to give this same speech again, I'll die. I look at those kids, who are always completely out of shape at the beginning, and want to tell them to go home and do something else, and so will I. Instead, I somehow get through the same motivational speech and appear very interested in their welfare. I probably should just quit at this point, because my heart is not in it anymore."

These are just a few examples of men like you, men who have learned how they need to act in order to continue earning a living. Since they can never share their real feelings with their clients, patients, customers, or bosses, it is important to be able to talk about them with the women in their lives. Don't shut her out, thinking she won't understand. She will. The comfort, understanding, and nurturing you'll get will give you the strength you need to get up every morning and earn a living.

## DON'T APOLOGIZE FOR A FEELING

Sometimes an apology for what you did is appropriate, but never apologize for what you felt. Feelings need to be recognized, shared, and aired. They are never right or wrong. They just are.

- I shouldn't feel so embarrassed.
- I shouldn't feel so uncomfortable.
- I shouldn't feel so defeated.

- I shouldn't feel so frustrated.
- I shouldn't feel so confused.
- I shouldn't feel so disappointed.
- I shouldn't feel so angry.
- I shouldn't feel so glad.

Don't ever "should" on your feelings. They are what they are. As I've said, you may have had parents who told you that you have no right to feel a certain way, but that's not true. You have every right to feel exactly how you do, and so does she.

That is the hard part, giving to another person what you never got yourself. So once again the question becomes, "Now that I'm getting new information, can I retrain myself in order to be a better mate?"

Whenever a woman comes to you with a feeling, whether it's fear, pain, disappointment, or embarrassment, the worst responses you can give are:

- You shouldn't feel that way.
- That's a dumb way to feel.
- I can't believe how you overreact to things.
- Why do you have to make mountains out of molehills?

Instead, just listen, then validate her feelings. Let her know in no uncertain terms that you care.

Once when I was at the airport, I overheard a girl telling her boyfriend that her foot was killing her, and she felt awful. I couldn't believe my ears when he responded, "Tell it to someone who cares."

This will be the same young man who'll shake his head

in shock when she finally breaks up with him. What needed to be said to her was, "Oh, you must feel awful. We have so much walking to do, and your foot is hurting. Here, let me get you a seat." If he had spent just three seconds of his time validating her feelings, she would have been comforted, and he would have had a secure place in her heart.

Have you ever seen a child crying, and the mother says, "Come here so I can kiss it and make it better"? The child stops crying immediately and actually feels better. This is the same principle. There are three understood messages that come with the kiss:

1. I hear what you're saying.
2. I understand what you're saying.
3. I want to comfort you.

The next time your mate is hurting, tell her to come here, and you'll kiss it and make it better. It works wonders and is a welcome change to hearing:

- Well, go take an aspirin.
- Quit complaining.
- If you think you're hurting, let me tell you about me.

These are certainly not statements that show you understand what she's feeling.

## DON'T BRING IT HOME

Some men make the mistake of bringing their frustrations on the job home with them. What a mistake! Imagine that you have two glasses of water in front of you. One is clear and represents your personal life, and the other is murky and represents your professional life. Why would you want to pour the dirty water into the glass with the clear, clean water? All you would end up with is two glasses of dirty water. Why not keep them separate? If your job doesn't fulfill your expectations and is a source of discontent, of course you should share your feelings about it, but don't take it out on the person you love. Don't bring it home that way. It's a decision you can make. Just because one part of your life isn't working right doesn't mean the other has to break down too. You can decide that you've done the best you can for eight hours a day, and now you will devote the rest of the day to expending all the attention and effort you have to making your loved one happy. "I will give her all that I am capable of giving."

Cal agreed that his mood at home was directly related to the kind of day he had at work. "No matter what she did, Samantha never could get me to change my moods, so she just stopped trying. When we were first married, she'd try to comfort me or say something humorous, but I just wanted to wallow in my gloom and frustration. Now, she hardly notices when I come home. She's usually busy doing something else. I guess it's not much fun being with someone who is grumpy, tired, and frustrated all the time, especially if you can never get them out of the mood they're in."

Take inventory of all the wonderful traits you possess, all

your strengths, and make the time you spend at home count every bit as much as the time you spend at work.

## ATTACK THE PROBLEM, NOT THE PERSON

Sometimes you think you know what you're feeling, but you are not exactly sure why you're feeling the way you do. Anger has always been an acceptable masculine trait. You may have seen your father throwing things, screaming obscenities, or using physical violence.

We tend to display behavior that is familiar to us. That's why statistics show that a child raised with violence and abuse tends to become a violent and abusive adult. What you saw as a child you tend to repeat as an adult unless you are willing to stop, think, and retrain yourself into reacting in a more positive, beneficial way. The next time you experience anger toward your mate, stop and think about what you're really feeling. This takes time and practice, but you can get really good at this.

Harold had a chance to practice this exercise as soon as he got home from class. He expected his wife to greet him and be eager to listen to what he had heard that day, but instead he came home to a woman who was engrossed in a conversation on the phone with her girlfriend. Harold's immediate reaction was anger.

He said, "My normal response would have been to say to my wife, 'Yak, yak, yak, that's all you ever do. You're nothing but a blabbermouth.' "

You can imagine how his evening would have ended.

Harold continued, "I stopped and thought about what I

was really feeling, and when she got off the phone, I told her that all the way home I had really been looking forward to talking about the class with her. I got so much out of the class, and I wanted to share it with her. I was so disappointed when I found her on the phone, because I had to wait for my turn to talk to her."

Janis responded, "Oh, sweetheart, I'm so sorry. Barbara called a few minutes ago, and it was long-distance. She was so upset because her son got an F on his report card. I tried to comfort her and get off as soon as I could. Sit down and tell me all about it. I really want to hear about everything that happened."

After that, they were able to enjoy each other's company, and they both went to bed happy, not angry.

Dennis said that most of the time he came home from work to a house that was a mess. The kids' toys were everywhere, beds were never made, and dishes were in the sink. He admitted to me privately that he had, on occasion, called his wife a slob. He always muttered under his breath loud enough for her to hear. Then he stopped and thought about his real feelings. He sat her down and told her how the untidiness of the house affected his self-worth.

He told her, "I really look forward to coming home, and somehow, if I knew you were also looking at the clock and were preparing for my arrival, then I'd feel so special. I feel so insignificant when you don't go out of your way to straighten things up. I'm so embarrassed about the way the house looks most of the time. Growing up, my mom was an alcoholic who often slept it off until three in the afternoon. I never brought friends home because I was so ashamed of where I lived. I don't like feeling the same way now. I know the kids are a handful, and you're doing your best, but maybe we could get you some part-time help so things would get a little easier for you."

Dennis said that the very next day he saw a remarkable change in his wife's behavior. Not only were the toys picked up, the dishes cleaned, and dinner ready, but there was music on, the kids were gone, and his wife, to his amazement, had gotten all dressed up for his arrival. She later told him that she would really try to put more effort into making him feel special, since he meant so much to her. She said that somewhere along the way, she had simply stopped being a wife and had gotten into the role of being only a mother.

Terry's arguments, for the past several months, centered around how much money his wife, Myrna, spent. Every time he got a MasterCard bill, he'd go into a tirade. He accused her of being a "rich witch," his favorite term, who didn't know the meaning of a dollar. She obviously had no shut-off valve, and he saw to it that her spending stopped. He took away her credit cards and checking account and began giving her an allowance. This marriage was going down the tubes fast! He was sensing her distance and the destruction of his marriage. During the "Light Her Fire" course, he really thought about his true feelings and decided to see if sharing them made a difference.

Terry asked Myrna out to dinner so they could talk and have an evening to themselves. When he explained that he wanted to talk about money, her immediate reaction was, "Look, all of a sudden you have become a stingy tightwad and care only about yourself. Are you going to ruin this dinner, too, and tell me what I can eat based on the prices?"

He felt his anger rise, but he forced himself to calm down and not react to her. He began by saying, "No, you can have anything you want on the entire menu, and if you don't see anything you like, I'll special order it. I don't care about the cost."

That calmed Myrna down instantly, and he began to sense her tenseness easing. She was then receptive to what he had to say. Terry began to explain that his company had announced that in the next few months there would be a large number of changes, one of which was to let many people go and force retirement for those who had been there for a long time. He told her, "Since I'm fifty years old, I'm one of the ones on the list for an early retirement. My boss confided in me in hopes that I could prepare myself for what is coming soon. I didn't want to tell you, because I didn't see the need for the two of us worrying about what the future holds. At my age, it won't be easy to find another job that pays as much as I'm getting now. I always thought I could continue to support you in the manner to which you are accustomed. Now I'm scared to death that without the money, you'll leave me and find a richer man."

Myrna sat shocked at what she was hearing. "Do you think I love you because of the things you've given me? I love you for who you are, not what we have! I'm so relieved to hear that this is the reason you've been so unbearable to live with lately. I thought there was another woman in your life, and you were going to spend your money on her and cut me out of your life. I figured you wanted to get me angry enough so that I would file for divorce. This is a situation I can handle. We don't need this big house now that the kids are all grown up. We can buy a small condo and pay cash with our equity in the house and have enough left over to live comfortably. I've been wanting to get a job for years so that I can feel better about myself. I have too much leisure time as it is. We'll work this out together."

Isn't that a great new start for Terry and Myrna? Most couples, like them, continually argue about things that have nothing to do with their real feelings until it is much too late.

I came from a family in which sleep was very precious. You walked on tiptoe and whispered if anyone was sleeping. Much to my shock, the first morning of our honeymoon, I felt a body close to mine and arms around me and my husband whispering that it was time to get up. I couldn't believe my ears. It was six-thirty, the middle of the night as far as I was concerned, especially since we'd been up until one o'clock. I'm like Snoopy, allergic to mornings.

So what does this wonderful new wife do? I proceed to yell at my husband, "How dare you wake me up while I'm sleeping! You are really inconsiderate, and I can't believe how selfish you are!"

In a very loving tone, he explained how he just couldn't wait to be with me. He had waited years to wake up beside me, cuddle, and then have breakfast together. "Besides," he added jokingly, "we'll have enough time to sleep when we're dead!"

My idea, of course, was to have brunch around noon, not breakfast at 7:00 A.M. As he turned over, I could sense his loneliness and rejection, so getting up in the middle of the night seemed like the only wifely thing to do. To this day, I force myself up on weekends many hours earlier than I would prefer. In defense of my husband, he stays up much later enjoying the night life than he would prefer, just to please me. Needless to say, because we love each other so much and want to fulfill each other's needs, we are a very tired—but happy—couple on weekends! Now, if I went back to our original honeymoon morning and he had reacted differently, I might never have had the understanding or desire to change my sleeping habits. If he had started calling me lazy or inconsiderate, I would have reacted with anger and certainly wouldn't have been responsive to his feelings.

So remember, if you have a bad temper and resort to name-calling, accusations, and blame, it's a sure bet that your mate will either ignore you, argue with you, or try to hurt you back in some way. On the other hand, if you take the time to stop, think about why you are angry, and then, in a loving way, reveal your true feelings, you'll have a woman who responds to you by being a more loving, understanding, and nurturing mate. It's not easy, but it will be well worth the extra effort.

## CONFLICT IS NECESSARY

Many couples claim that they never argue. In fact, when they finally split up or get a divorce, everyone is astonished, and the general comment is, "I don't believe it. Dale and Leesa seemed so happy. They never disagreed about anything!"

I can't tell you how many times a wife or husband comes to my class completely dismayed that their mate has left. They say that there were no clues. You've heard the story, I'm sure, about the husband who went out to get some milk and never came back. I can assure you that if two people never argue, it means that at least one person in the relationship never expresses feelings. Nothing can be more damaging to you and your relationship than suppressing your feelings. It's like covering a hand grenade with a silk scarf to keep it from exploding.

Conflict leads to growth; it does not have to lead to divorce. It is impossible to find two people who will agree entirely about everything. Arguing is a healthy and necessary method of resolving tension that exists between two people who have different personalities, viewpoints, ways of doing things, and different sets of priorities.

Anger is nothing more than a more basic feeling of hurt, disappointment, worry, fear, or embarrassment that is being covered up. It is only through conflict and arguments that two people can understand the other's point of view and ultimately reach some kind of compromise. In this process, you'll find there is not only personal growth, but also more intimacy and sensuality between the two of you.

Many students of mine are shocked to find out what my neighbors already know: my husband and I argue all the time. In our twenty-four years together, I'm sure many windows have been closed by neighbors not wanting to listen to us venting our anger. (For others, we've probably provided an evening's entertainment!) Both of us are extremely strong-willed and opinionated. Maybe the fact that we were both the oldest children in our families has something to do with that. We don't suppress any hostility. It comes right out, is dealt with, and then it's over. There is no harboring of resentment or pretense when one of us is annoyed with the other.

I will admit that as we've gotten older and a little more

tired, we've gotten better at seeing each other's point of view more quickly, and arguments that used to last for hours are over much faster. At the end of every disagreement, we always have new insight or information, along with that wonderful feeling of closeness that comes with the joy of making up.

Harry, who has been happily married for seventeen years to Rhonda, said, "We are experts when it comes to arguments. We used to argue about everything. She'd get upset when I dropped my pants on the floor, at the hair I left in the sink after shaving, at not calling if I was going to be late, at my making social appointments without consulting her, and when I changed the TV channels while she was watching a show. I found her neatness and strong emotions annoying. But you know, our arguments never lasted very long, and through the years, we both know where we stand and have a greater respect for one another."

This kind of relationship is so much less fragile than one in which the husband and wife pretend not to be annoyed or not to disagree. Couples who air their feelings have a better chance to gain insight into their relationship and respect for each other. Most important, their sex lives won't be affected by taking hidden anger to bed with them. Those couples that don't argue, but experience long periods of silence instead, are really arguing without words. Although there is no noise going on outside the bedroom, there's also a very good chance that there will be no noise inside the bedroom either.

Stan decided that it was time to deal with the conflict in his marriage that he had been avoiding for years. "I always felt that my wife, who works part time as a nurse, should shoulder more responsibilities around the house. Since I was working full time, and she was putting in only four hours a day, I did not think I should have to do household chores and take care of the kids at night. It was the only time I had to relax. My reasoning was that whoever makes the most money during the day deserves some peace and quiet at night. Every time Dorothy complained or got upset at the amount of work she had to do, I'd just tune her out. I knew she always seemed tired and never responded to me sexually, but I just figured that was the way she was, and I was stuck with it.

"One night after your class, I went home and told Dorothy that we really needed to talk. I wanted to hear her point of view, and I promised her I wouldn't blow up. She explained that yes, she was putting in only four hours at work, but she was also putting in ten hours at home, cooking, cleaning, and taking care of the kids. That was a total of fourteen hours a day, compared to my eight. She said she didn't feel like a woman anymore, only a maid. We spent most of that evening talking, and I decided that she really did need my help. Since then, I've been doing my part, and Dorothy is a different woman. She says I've added two hours to her life every day, and she's going to see to it that she makes good use of them, showering me with affection."

Brian never wanted to argue, because he didn't see any point to it. The fact that Anita was working late every evening was bothering him, but he was not the type of man who wanted any conflict. After learning about how conflict can lead to new insight and growth, he decided it was time to try it out.

He said that he just blurted out one night, "I can't stand

you working late anymore. You spend more time with your boss than you do with me."

Anita's immediate reaction was anger. "How dare you feel that way!" she yelled. "I'm just trying to get my work done, and besides, my boss needs me!"

When Brian finally admitted that he was lonely and needed her, too, they arrived at an agreement. Anita said she'd tell her boss that she could work late only one night a week; she needed to spend the rest of her evenings with her husband. Brian also revealed, with a smile on his face, that the night after they finally got down to how neglected he was feeling, they had the best night of lovemaking they'd had in a long time.

## TAKE CARE, NOT ADVANTAGE

Neither partner ever wants to be taken advantage of or taken for granted. It's only human nature to try to take advantage of another person's generosity or easygoing nature. Pay particular attention to this tendency, and be sure that neither of you is doing it.

If you had a secretary who was coming in weekends and staying late at night to complete the work you gave her, not too many bosses would say, "You know, you've been working too hard. Why don't you say no to me once in a while and work less?" Your tendency would be to keep giving her more work. And you'll change only if she tells you she's overworked and underpaid. It's only then that you begin to recognize her as a human being and not a machine.

It is also human nature to take for granted that once a

person falls in love with you, it will be forever. When a woman finally says "I hate you," that's when you learn that feelings can fluctuate from day to day. If either of you keeps those bad feelings inside, the bad slowly overtakes the good. It's only after she's gone that you remember why you were there in the first place. Conflict makes us stop and think. You may not realize immediately that your behavior has affected her in a negative way, but the more she stands her ground, the more you are forced to stop and think about her and her feelings.

Take care to acknowledge her feelings and express your own to her. Tell her your troubles and listen to hers, and remember, it's okay not to agree about everything. If you live alone, you don't have to deal with any conflict, and you certainly don't have anyone with whom to argue. But if you live with another person, it's important to understand that conflict will be part of your lives. Welcome it, learn from it, and grow from it.

## ACTION ASSIGNMENT #4

1. Begin to pay attention to your own feelings as well as to your mate's. Whenever you feel any anger or resentment, stop, think about what you're really feeling, and then explain your true feelings to her. Don't build up resentment by postponing your needs for a more convenient time.
2. Set aside one evening this week and ask your mate to participate in this assignment. Each of you write a ten-statement biography. If someone had to understand the

*real* you, what ten important things would they need to know? Reveal the person beneath the mask you wear. Reveal your honest feelings, as opposed to superficial appearances. For example:

1) I am terrified of getting old.
2) The turning point in my life was when my father died.
3) I'm afraid of rejection.
4) It means so much to me for you to love me and for me to be special to you.
5) I'm afraid of being a failure.
6) It's hard for me to ask for help.
7) I feel trapped at my job.
8) I appear strong at work, but many times it's only a facade.
9) I want to be physically attractive to you.
10) I feel as if I should be a much better father and spend more time with the children.

3. Make every attempt this week to leave your work-related worries and frustrations at the office. Plan to greet your mate with enthusiasm, and concentrate on giving her your best.

Dear Ellen,

No one can believe the change that has occurred in me. I've gone from being depressed and insecure most of the time to being the woman I've always wanted to be, radiating confidence and happiness. I find I'm joking and laughing all the time. It's like a black cloud has lifted and allowed the sunshine to come out. Someone at work actually asked me if I was pregnant, because she's always seen that glow on a woman during that time in her life. I laughed and said, "I am definitely not pregnant, just content and very happy." It all comes from the new atmosphere in our home. Herbert has become such a positive husband. He has more peace and harmony than I've ever seen him have before. I can't stop thinking how lucky we were to find out about your class.

Love,
Sue

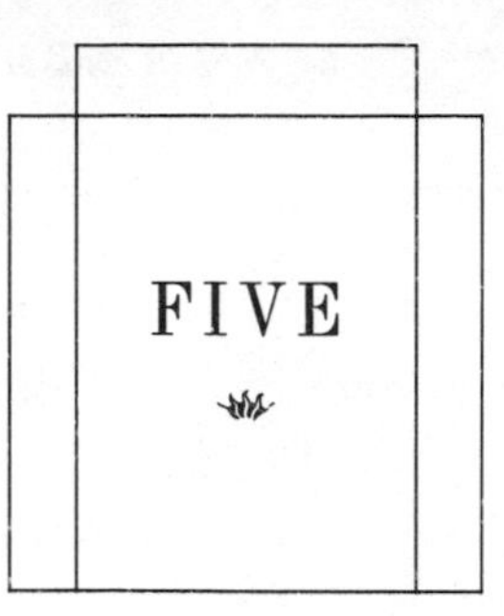

# FIVE

# *Turn-ons, Turn-offs*

## A GOOD, HARD LOOK AT YOURSELF

I asked the women in my classes to list the top fifteen traits that turned them off to men, then to list the top fifteen traits that they considered turn-ons. But remember, if you don't pay close attention to what turns her off, you'll never get the chance to turn her on.

| TURN-OFFS | TURN-ONS |
|---|---|
| Lack of self-esteem | Confidence |
| Laziness | Sense of humor |
| Lack of humor | Intelligence |
| Lack of confidence | Support |
| Lack of goals | Sensitivity |
| Lack of understanding | Self-worth |
| Lack of tenderness | Goals |
| Negativity | Imagination |
| Self-centeredness | Independence |
| Extreme jealousy | Desire |

| TURN-OFFS | TURN-ONS |
|---|---|
| Insecurity | Courage |
| Smothering dependence | Compassion |
| Self-pity | Decisiveness |
| Lack of trust | Sense of integrity |
| No ambition | Dignity |

Use these turn-ons and turn-offs as a guide to increase your awareness of yourself and to enhance your personal growth. Not only will you be able to turn your mate on, but you will feel better about yourself in the process.

## AN INWARD JOURNEY

No one I know enjoys being rejected, ignored, disappointed, or pushed aside for a more suitable mate, yet it is these very reactions from the significant people in your life that force you to look inside yourself and ultimately to stretch, grow, and gain more knowledge and understanding about yourself.

Falling in love is the easy part. It is effortless and pleasurable. Staying in love is the ultimate challenge. It takes effort, time, concentration, knowledge, and commitment. Oddly enough, these are the same ingredients necessary to be successful in your professional life. The easy part is getting a job. The hard part is fulfilling the requirements that are necessary to remain employed.

I always ask the men in my class to declare whether they feel they are steel, velvet, or a combination of both. Of thirty-five men, approximately fifteen usually define themselves as steel, the other fifteen as velvet, and the remaining five feel they are a combination of both. In the weeks that follow, it becomes apparent to everyone that those who possess both traits are not only more able to satisfy women, but are ultimately the most self-actualized, fulfilled men in general.

Let's begin your inward journey together and develop both your steel and velvet qualities so you can become more of the man you already are. If you can combine the strength of a lion or tiger with the gentleness of a teddy bear or pussycat, if you can be as hard as a rock and as soft as drifting fog, you can become the most sought-after man on earth.

## TURNING A WOMAN OFF

It's important to start with observing the turn-offs, because, as I said earlier, if you are not aware of the results that negative behavior has, you'll never get the opportunity to show your mate what a terrific man you really are.

### INDECISIVENESS

No woman likes a wishy-washy man. If she asks him if he wants to go to a movie next Saturday night, Mr. Wishy-Washy says, "We'll see" or "Maybe." If she asks him what restaurant he wants to eat at or what kind of food he's in the mood for, he replies, "I don't care" or "It makes no difference to me." If she asks him where he would like to go for a vacation, his response is, "It's up to you."

Brad described his indecisive behavior in this way: "I'm very easygoing, and I'm sure that's one of the reasons Mandy fell in love with me. I was beginning, however, to drive her crazy. I never expressed any opinions of my own and certainly never made any decisions, minor or major. My usual response was, 'Anything you want, dear, will be just fine with me.' I'm sure Mandy wanted to slug me sometimes. She must have felt as if she were by herself, with this excess baggage in the house—me. She told me that just once, she'd like to have a good argument over different viewpoints or decisions. After Ellen's class, I began giving her my opinion, and I made an effort to be more decisive. I really feel better about myself, and I think Mandy has found a new respect for me."

Another thing that can drive a woman crazy is a man who constantly asks questions. Even teen-age girls will say they hate it when a boy calls for a date and starts with, "Are you busy Saturday night?" We all know why he asks, of course. If she says she's not busy, then he doesn't feel like a fool asking her out. If she says she is busy, then he can change the subject quickly.

But a girl would much rather hear, "I'd like to take you out Saturday night, that is, of course, if you're not busy."

I know it seems like a minor difference, but the girl will immediately respect his risking making a statement rather than asking a question. Besides, when he asks if she's busy, she feels foolish saying no. To her, it means "No, I have nothing to do, because I'm not popular," or "No, because no one else has asked me out."

Often, when a man asks a question instead of expressing a desire, the woman's unspoken response is, "If he has to ask, then the answer is no."

"Can I kiss you?" could be replaced with "I'd like to kiss you."

"Do you want me to buy you a present?" could be changed to "I'm going to buy you a present." (Even if she says no, she always means yes in this case.)

Many times you really don't care, and just want to please your mate, but if she has to make all the decisions, eventually it adds up to too much responsibility on her part, which results in a loss of respect for you.

## CONTROL

Some men feel that they should make all the decisions. These are the men of steel, they proudly proclaim. There's a big difference between living with a man who possesses that wonderful steel quality and who is also a democratic leader, with his mate as his chief advisor, and living with a tyrant.

Alfred was one of those men who volunteered to share his new insight. "I was the tyrant Ellen has told us about. I treated my wife like a puppet, and I pulled all the strings. I decided when it was time to have children, picked the house we lived in, chose the car we drove, and selected the friends we would spend time with. I controlled everything. I chose when and where we had vacations, the kind of food I wanted her to cook, and I was the one who decided when, where, and how we would have sex.

"Yolanda was only nineteen when I married her, and I was twenty-nine. Her father deserted her mother when she was very young, so she welcomed my take-charge personality. I guess I enjoyed being the father she never had, but the novelty wore off years ago for her. Now she's thirty-five, and she constantly tells me how she would like more respect in our marriage, that she wants a partnership, not a dictatorship. I finally see that unless I start taking her opinions, needs, and thoughts into consideration and learn the art of negotiation, I'm heading for big trouble."

When a man states his opinions or makes decisions that he feels are beneficial, he should never forget to add, "What do you think?" or "What would you like?" He must also be willing to change his original plans some of the time. It's part of the loving act called compromise.

## SABOTAGE

Terrence said that he blew up when his wife, Claire, decided that she wanted to go back to school and get a degree in teaching. "I growled at her, saying, 'Fine, go ahead. You'll probably flunk anyway. You never were a good student.' To make matters worse, I told her that I didn't know what she was trying to prove. Didn't she think I was earning enough money around here? I added that I wasn't going to help one bit while she was out playing student. I kept that promise, and Claire had all the children's activities to attend, plus the household chores. She never had time to study. I really thought that if I kept her 'barefoot and pregnant,' I'd have a loyal wife. To be honest, I was afraid that she would outgrow me. Before 'Light Her Fire,' no one ever told me that if I took her needs into consideration and helped her achieve personal growth, she'd love me even more. As it turned out, she got an F in one class and two

D's in the others. I don't have to tell you how she feels about herself now. If it takes the rest of my life, I'm going to encourage her to try again, but this time with my help."

Martin told us that his wife was overweight for her five-foot-two-inch frame and was trying to stick to a diet. "I'm guilty of sabotaging Adriana," he said. "I would bring home cookies and ice cream and tell her that since she would only lose the weight for a short time anyway, why torture herself? I would do my best to convince her that she had no willpower as I dished out the ice cream. The truth is that underneath it all, I was afraid that if she did lose all that weight, she would leave me and find somebody else. I guess I never considered the possibility that she might love me more if I supported her when she set goals for herself and encouraged her to achieve them."

Terrence and Martin have both realized that with their wives' personal fulfillment could come a deeper, more passionate love for the man who helped make it all possible.

## JEALOUSY

Some men think that jealousy is proof of their love. In reality, it is proof of insecurity, and an insecure man is very unattractive to women. Some jealousy is normal in any love relationship. Every man wants daily reminders that his mate won't find greener pastures, outgrow him, or find other people or activities that are more exciting and interesting than he is.

But extreme jealousy will eventually ruin a perfectly good relationship. If a woman has friends, interests, obligations, and activities that take time away from you, it is your constant accusations that will drive her away, not those other people, interests, or activities.

When two people love each other, there has to be trust between them. It's quite normal for you to want her to account for her time away from you. These are questions that you can ask her and expect to get honest answers.

"How come you're home so late?"
"Who was there at the party?"
"Anything interesting happen today?"

When she answers them as openly and honestly as she can, it's not appropriate to call her a liar or sarcastically say, "Yeah, sure, now tell me the truth," or "Who did you flirt with?" or "How many guys tried to pick you up?" Questions such as these begin to attack your mate's integrity. It is also normal for her to assume that if you are so unsure of her feelings for you, maybe *you* are the one she needs to worry about. Why would you even think she's flirting unless maybe that's what you do when she's not around? Why would you think someone's trying to pick her up unless possibly that's what you do?

Chad saw immediately the grief he was causing his girlfriend. "Every day, I give Rebecca the third degree. It's as if I'm a drill sergeant, and she's a new recruit. She keeps telling me that she might as well have an affair with someone else, because no matter what she says, I never believe her anyway. My way of dealing with my jealousy is prolonged silence and anger, even though deep down I know that she's not guilty of anything. I see now that if I don't stop this, my fear will become a reality. After all, she's getting the same punishment she would if she were fooling around with other guys. It's my insecurity that will drive her away from me, not another man."

## BLAMING AND COMPLAINING

Men who don't take responsibility for their own lives need an alibi to explain why they are so unhappy or unfulfilled. They spend most of their time and energy blaming other people, events, or things for their inadequacies or misfortunes, complaining about them instead of making the best of them. They've developed a great list of excuses.

- *Parents*—If only I had better parents.
- *Wife*—If only I had a more supportive wife.
- *Boss*—If only I had a better boss.
- *The economy*—If only we didn't have inflation and high taxes.
- *Health*—If only I weren't so sick.
- *Physical appearance*—If only I were better-looking.
- *Mental ability*—If only I were smarter.
- *Age*—If only I were younger.
- *Personality*—If only I weren't so shy.
- *Fate*—If only I were luckier.

Boy, that's a great list to choose from, isn't it? Who could argue with all those alibis, all those "if onlys"?

I'll tell you who. Anyone who has ever accomplished anything in his life in spite of his shortcomings. Roosevelt could have used his health as an excuse not to run for president. Kennedy could have used his religion as an excuse not to run for president. Truman could have used his lack of a college education as an excuse.

You don't have to consider running for president of the United States, but I would like you to spend less time blaming things over which you have no control and start concentrating on taking charge of your own life. It's too depressing for a woman to live with someone who is always complaining.

Leon explained that he was one of those men who always come home complaining and blaming anything or anyone for his awful day. "It's as if I'm the flat tire, and Jean is the pump. She always tries so hard to pump me up. That poor, sweet woman! No wonder she's become hostile toward me. Who's there to pump her up? I think I'm going to try looking in the mirror and place some of that blame where it ought to be."

Cheryl revealed her frustration with Ray, who is always in a bad mood when he comes home. "The whole family walks on eggshells when Ray walks through the door. He's always upset at the traffic and how long it took him to get home. He'll start cursing at the kids for leaving their bikes outside the garage or their toys in the hallway. The house is never clean or neat enough, no matter how hard I try, and he usually complains about whatever I've made for dinner. Heaven forbid that I should get a phone call before or after dinner and take away time from listening to him moan and groan. He's annoyed all evening at the kids, who want to talk about 'nonsense,' as he calls it. They're only five and seven, and he makes it quite obvious how bored he is with their chatter. He's critical about how I handle things and always tells me how it should have been done differently."

After taking my class for men, Ray began to see that although he couldn't change some of the irritating little things that happen to all of us daily, he could change the way he looked at them, and he certainly had control over his reactions to them.

"I bought a set of motivational tapes to listen to while I was stuck in traffic," he said. "This calmed me down considerably. I also decided that I would try to notice all the things Cheryl did to please me and give her compliments instead of criticism. I realized that her phone calls were important, because sometimes they were her only means of outside stimulation. After all, she was with the kids all day long. Most of all, I finally appreciated having those wonderful kids and a woman who really cared about me."

You, too, can make the decision to improve the quality of your life. If you take a positive attitude toward the people, events, and things in your life, you'll find little to blame and even less to complain about.

## SELF-IMPORTANCE

Women are turned off by men who are too wrapped up with their own self-importance. These men never stop talking about themselves. They'll spend hours recounting their day, their goals, their ideas, and their accomplishments and never once ask a question about their mates.

Once, in one of the women's classes, everybody was eager to hear about Julie's date, because the previous week she had told us that she had met the most gorgeous man while waiting to have her car repaired. They had talked for only a few minutes, and he had asked for her phone number. He called, and she was so excited about seeing him that Saturday night.

We were all disappointed as Julie said, "Forget him! All he talked about all night was himself. For five hours, he never took a breath. I felt like I could have left, gone shopping, come back, and he wouldn't have known the difference. As it turned out, after the first two hours, I just turned off and really didn't listen for the rest of the evening. Not once did he ask me anything about myself. What an egomaniac!"

Felix, who is a doctor, admitted that he, too, was wrapped up in himself. "I work in the emergency room of a large hospital. When I come home, I usually make it very clear that I'm not interested in hearing the trivial matters Tammy has to deal with as a full-time housewife. I've always felt that my work was so much more important than what she does. I realize now that while saving lives every day is important, shaping the lives of our children has just as much value as my profession."

When a man puts a higher value on himself and what he does than on the woman in his life, he is automatically sending out the message, "You are not the one who's important. I am."

If you are not willing to listen to how many dirty diapers she's changed and how many times the baby burped, you will eventually stop hearing about everything else she considers important, and most of all, she'll stop listening to you, too. There is a saying, "Nobody cares how much you know until they know how much you care."

When a man comes home late and hasn't bothered to call, the issue is not the dinner that was waiting. It's the feeling of worthlessness that his woman feels that is the issue. If you had an appointment with a client in business and you couldn't get there at your appointed time, you'd call and let him know. Does the most important person in your life deserve less? A man who places a high importance on his mate gives her the courtesy of a phone call to let her know he won't be home on time. If your excuse is "I was in the middle of a meeting," you are still making a decision that the people you are meeting with are more important than your mate. A woman wants to be treated with the same consideration you would give any VIP, and she deserves no less.

## ALL WORK AND NO PLAY

All work and no play not only makes Jack a dull boy, but also a boring mate. Ambition is definitely one of the traits in a man that women find attractive, and for good reason. Ambition can lead to money, power, and sometimes even fame. But women who wind up with an ambitious workaholic are usually very lonely and find the price they pay is too high. The yacht they own is never used, the vacation home remains empty, and the clothes and jewels are never seen by their absentee husbands.

In the beginning, some men see their self-worth only in terms of the money they've earned. Eventually they learn that unless they can balance their earning power with their "playing" power, they will lose their family, friends, and, most important, themselves.

- Take time out to watch a sunrise or sunset.
- Take time off to go on a vacation.
- Take time off to take a lesson together. Sailing, golf, tennis, and horseback riding are just a few examples.
- Take time to appreciate the beauty in nature. Take a walk on the beach or in the woods.
- Take time to sit on the grass.
- Take time to stop and smell a flower.
- Take time to listen to birds sing.
- Take time to listen to the wind blow.
- Take time to feel the warm sunshine.

Give yourself permission to relax, retreat from daily obligations, and daydream. It will not only balance all that ambition you have, it will enhance it.

Jake, a successful businessman in his late sixties who came to class in search of some answers as to why his wife of forty-six years left him, sadly admitted, "I should have been a better husband and father. I wish I hadn't taken most of my life so seriously. I should have played harder and worked less."

While you still have choices, decide to create a more balanced life so that you will have few regrets. This means you'll have to stop every once in a while and watch that sunset hand in hand with the most important person in your life.

## NEEDING TO LOVE

Some men have taken my course because they can't seem to hold a woman's interest for very long. These men have been "dumped" repeatedly by women who chose a more suitable mate. Having been rejected many times, they are often in much emotional pain.

Randy stayed after class to seek some advice. "I don't understand why Jane wants to be my friend. I've heard that line more times than I'd like to admit. The other one I always hear is that it's not me, it's her. I did everything I could to please her, and now she wants out."

It was evident that Randy *needed* to be in a relationship. That was his problem. There's a big difference in choosing to be in a relationship and needing to be in one. Desperation is a turn-off to most women. She wants to know that you are a complete human being, with or without her, and not dependent on her to make you feel whole. When you have developed your own goals, interests, and views, she gets turned on to the prospect of having a man she respects. When a man does everything he does because he is desperately trying to please a woman, he either has not developed himself or has given up on himself in order to be loved by her.

It is human nature to want what we can't have. What we can have anytime, anywhere, is much less desirable than that elusive something that is just out of reach. A nonchalant attitude is sometimes exactly what is needed in the beginning of a relationship.

But let me tell you about Randy's happy ending. He called Jane and left her with these words: "Look, I know I'm the best thing that ever happened to you, and if you can't see that, well, that's too bad." Then he began dating again. He adopted a more relaxed, casual attitude and found that many women were attracted to him and eager to pursue a relationship. One month later, he received a phone call at work from Jane. She told him she couldn't stand it any longer. She never realized what she had until she lost it. She wanted to get back together, and he told her he'd have to think about it. "It was the greatest feeling on earth to see her come to this conclusion all on her own while I was having a good time," he said. One year later, I received their wedding announcement.

There's a wonderful quote I have hanging in my classroom: "If you love someone, set them free. If they come back, it was meant to be." If you are a man who is needy and dependent, you are going to have to learn to act independent and confident. What may start out as an act will become part of you as you see the results of this behavior. You have to come across as a person who can live with or without her.

No matter how strong, successful, and independent a woman is, she is still looking for a man she can respect, look up to, and admire. In her search for an assertive man, she will test your limits. If you don't have any, because you're afraid of losing her, then she will walk all over you. Once she sees you as weak, predictable, dependent, and needy, all chances for romance with this woman stops.

Debra told the class about how her romantic feelings toward Mel turned into friendship. "I met Mel at the company where I work. I was instantly attracted to his sense of humor and his independence. I was twenty-two years old, still living at home, and Mel had his own apartment. The turning point in our relationship came when I had to go out of town for two weeks to complete a business transaction. Mel literally fell apart in front of my eyes. He started whining about how I'd probably meet someone else while I was away. He also kept telling me how he could not function while I was gone. He begged me to tell our boss that I couldn't go. All of a sudden I saw this frail, sad individual who was making such a big deal over nothing. I finally left, and he called me at least three times a day where I was working and left at least two messages for me when I returned to my hotel. I dreaded coming home at the end of the two weeks. I finally got up the nerve to tell him that I just wasn't ready for a serious relationship with him."

Mel should have pretended that he would have been just fine without her. Debra would not have lost respect for him if he had just said, "I'm sure going to miss you, but two weeks will be up before you know it, and you'll be back in my arms again." He could have gone out of his way to contact friends and do things with them. When he did call, he could have told her about his activities. She would have felt a little twinge of jealousy that he was having so much fun without her, and she would not have been able to wait to get back to him.

## INSENSITIVITY

You may have seen him, in restaurants, in shops, in parking lots, the man who compromises the woman he is with by touching her in a way that she should never be subjected to in public. Intimate touching should only be done on intimate terms, at intimate times, and in an intimate setting. Women unanimously agree that they can't stand when a man grabs at their "private parts." To tell you the truth, I was amazed to find out how many women endure this kind of behavior from the men in their lives.

Erica explained how much she cared for her fiancé, but his actions in public were upsetting her. "We'd be going up an escalator, and he'd grab my rear end and squeeze it. Even though I would tell him to stop it, he would just laugh. I know it may sound crazy, but I actually began avoiding going to a mall where there was an escalator. But that didn't stop him. We'd be out with another couple, and out of the blue, he'd squeeze my breasts right in front of them. I'd die of embarrassment, and he'd just stand there with a smirk on his face. He didn't care where we were or how many people were around when he'd pinch and poke at intimate parts of my body. I tried to tell him how I felt and asked how he'd like it. You know what his response was? 'Go ahead, I'd love it! Make me a sex object and see how much I'd object.' "

Here's another difference between men and women. Women hate to be treated as sex objects, while men sometimes fantasize about it. To a woman, it's the ultimate insult. True love doesn't embarrass or humiliate the person you're with. If what you're doing to her is really what you'd like done to you, respect that she has different needs and different turn-ons. Respect her wishes as you would want her to respect yours. If you were a man who objected to your wife dressing in a provocative manner in public, and she ignored your feelings, you'd be embarrassed to be with her. There is not a woman alive who does not want the world to know that the man she is with respects her. You have to find out what feels good to her and what doesn't and adjust your actions accordingly. That's a sign of a good lover.

If you haven't recognized a part of yourself in any of these men, you deserve to be congratulated. If you have, rest assured that you can change these kinds of behavior overnight. By recognizing them and admitting that you might have some of these traits, you have taken the first step toward becoming the world's greatest lover.

Creating a perfect balance between strength and tenderness is usually not a talent most men are born with. It takes time to develop, but it's a goal you can continually strive to obtain. By carefully observing the reactions your mate has to your behavior, you'll get a clearer picture of which part you need to concentrate on more.

## TURNING A WOMAN ON

Now let's look at some of the great turn-ons. Pay particular attention to these traits and cultivate them in yourself. You'll not only turn her on like you wouldn't believe, you'll like yourself better, too!

### RADIATING CONFIDENCE

Have you ever thought your looks are what's keeping you from having a woman love you? Well, you're wrong. *Handsome is in the eye of the beholder.*

When I've asked women to list the traits in a man that

they thought were important, number one on almost everyone's list was confidence. A man who knows who he is and feels good about himself wins hands-down every time. It's not how you look that turns women off, it's how you act that does it. Handsome is as handsome does.

If you think you're too short, too tall, too bald, your ears are too large, your eyes are no good, or whatever other physical trait you think is inadequate, then consider some of the world's most sought-after men, past and present. Woody Allen, Carlo Ponti, Gene Wilder, Telly Savalas, Michael Tucker, Henry Kissinger, Dudley Moore, and Danny DeVito have never had any problem attracting women. Not all women are looking for a Tom Selleck look-alike or an Arnold Schwarzenegger body.

Lisa summed it up one night, and most of the women in the class nodded in agreement. "A truly sexy man is one who likes himself and knows how to treat a woman with respect, understanding, and kindness."

## A SENSE OF HUMOR

What would we do without a sense of humor? Humor can see us through the worst of times and make the good times even better. For most women, a sense of humor is one of the most valuable traits a man can possess.

Years ago, I had a friend help me lighten my hair and I had an allergic reaction to the bleaching solution. She immediately rushed me to the hospital just as I was, with the bleach still in my hair. As a result, the bleach was in much longer than it should have been, and my hair was bright orange for months. My husband was very sympathetic and took good care of me. One day he said, "You know, it's not so bad. You've always acted like a 'Lucy,' and now you look like her." He called me Lucy for weeks, and you know, I didn't mind. My husband has a very funny, wry sense of humor, and that's one of the reasons I fell in love with him. He has always made me laugh, especially when a sense of humor is needed in a particularly upsetting situation.

Many times, the element of surprise is very funny. Mason said that one night he decided to change his position in bed one hundred and eighty degrees. He put his feet where his head would normally be and his head where his feet usually were. His wife came from the bathroom into the dark bedroom and climbed into bed just as she did every night and talked to him a little. Then she rolled over, thinking she would snuggle up to his warm chest, but instead she found herself embracing a foot. She was still giggling when she got up the next morning.

Wade walked into the bedroom completely naked with a paper bag over his head. In a serious tone he asked his wife, "Would you still recognize me if you couldn't see my face?" "Alicia just cracked up," he told the class. "She couldn't stop laughing for at least an hour."

Murray was able to begin Jana's day with a smile. As soon as the alarm rang, he climbed over her to get out of bed. When she asked what he was doing, he said that every day he got out of bed on the left side, which was very lonely. Today, he decided he wanted to get up on the right side, where it wasn't so lonely. Jana laughed and told me she thought about it the whole day.

These examples are funny because of the spirit in which

they're given. But there is a big difference between that kind of humor and a cutting remark that is cruel and insensitive.

Donald explained that before "Light Her Fire," Jill was usually the brunt of his jokes. "I'd poke fun at her cooking, driving, interests, and anything else I could think of when we were around other people. Now I realize that what I was doing was really mean." He said that the previous Saturday night, they had had friends over, and he had consciously passed up something that before would have been the brunt of some cruel joke. "Jill had taken a class on ESP," he said. "Our friends seemed very interested in what she was saying about it, and instead of doing my usual, which would have been something like, 'Yeah, next week we're going to put her on *The Twilight Zone,*' I put my arm around her while she was talking. When she finished, I said, 'I'm really proud that Jill has learned so much.' She beamed and gave me a kiss on the cheek. Later, she told me how surprised she was that I hadn't made fun of her. What she didn't know was that I had decided I was never going to do that to her again."

Here are some guidelines to use in judging whether something is funny or not.

- It's funny if you're sure it's something she's not sensitive about.
- It's funny if you are not making fun of her weaknesses.
- It's funny if it doesn't cause her pain.
- It's funny if you're not revealing something she told you in confidence.
- It's funny if it doesn't humiliate her.

## LEAN ON ME

Never is the steel and velvet combination more important than in times of stress. A woman needs a man she can count on to be there for her, someone she can lean on. It's important to her that you be her friend as well as her lover.

Some men are so uncomfortable when their mates experience illness, the death of a loved one, or some other tragedy, that they take the easy way out when such emergencies arise. They choose not to deal with the problems and find excuses to disappear, either mentally or physically. Nothing can disappoint a woman more. The respect she once had disappears. If you're in a long-term relationship, you can bet that sooner or later some unforeseen event will wreak havoc in your mate's life.

Simon said that this part of the class had the most impact on him. "My wife's mother passed away three weeks ago," he began. "Janine was very close to her, and when she died unexpectedly in a car accident, Janine was despondent and utterly confused. I am an orphan. I spent my childhood in a series of foster homes, which taught me to depend only on myself. I tend to be rather aloof, and I get very uncomfortable at public displays of emotion. I guess it comes from years of keeping my own emotions buried in order not to feel pain. If I hadn't taken this class, my response to my wife's grief would have been to convince her just to make the funeral arrangements, call the rest of the family, and 'for heaven's sake, pull yourself together!'

"Instead, I concentrated on what she was going through and respected the fact that she had a right to her feelings, even if they were different from mine. I did my best to help her through this terrible time. At the funeral, instead of telling her to get hold of herself, I just held her and kept telling her over and over that I loved her and that I was there for her and would be forever. She's since told me how she will never forget how wonderful I was and what a difference I made. She told me she doesn't know what she would have done without me."

Phillip said he was really ashamed of his past behavior, but he was willing to share it with the hope that other men would not do as he had. "My wife, Penny, had a miscarriage a few years ago and had to go to the hospital. When she tried to get hold of me, my secretary said she didn't know where I was. It was nine o'clock by the time I got home, and I was completely exhausted. There was a message on the answering machine from the hospital. I called, and they told me she was in recovery and sleeping, so I decided to wait until morning to call her. The truth was that I hated hospitals and couldn't stand the thought of going there.

"The next morning when I called her, she really let me have it. I told her that I had felt she was in good hands. There was nothing I could have done to help. She tried to explain that she needed me to be there for moral support, not medical assistance. Things haven't been the same between us since that time. She has been polite, but distant. We just found out that she is pregnant again. The other night, I promised her that I would be there for her this time and told her what a fool I had been. I also agreed to go to childbirth classes and to be in the delivery room, two things I had adamantly opposed before. The sparkle in her eyes and the look on her face were worth putting her needs ahead of mine. It's been years since I felt that closeness, and

I'm not ever going to do anything to jeopardize her love for me again."

I have undergone several operations and can't imagine waking up and not seeing my husband there holding my hand and comforting me. He, too, hates hospitals (I'd guess most people feel that way to some degree), but his love and concern for my welfare have always been stronger than the discomfort he feels in a hospital setting.

When my mother died, I don't know what I would have done if he hadn't taken charge of making all the arrangements. Since I was distraught it was wonderful to have someone who was thinking clearly. It was the day before Christmas Eve, and it was not easy to get a flight to Florida. He went straight to a travel agent and paid full fare, it being a last-minute reservation. Never once did he complain about the price (which he normally would do) or the inconvenience of his having to take care of the household while I was gone.

When a crisis occurs, a ray of sunshine through the dark clouds is a man who says:

"Honey, I'm here for you."
"Sweetheart, don't worry, I'll take care of everything."
"Darling, you can count on my help."
"Sweetheart, *lean on me.*"

Of course, there is a flip side to that coin. When tragedy or disappointment strikes you, allow her the pleasure of comforting you. A relationship is give and take, and a man who always portrays that stiff upper lip is not one a woman can get close to. The ability to show your feelings is the velvet characteristic that women feel is necessary in order to have an intimate relationship with a man. Remember minister and author Robert Schuller's famous words, "Tough times never last; tough people do." And here's another well-known saying: "When the going gets tough, the tough get going." Sometimes, the toughest thing you can do is to show that you care.

## SUPPORT

A truly confident man is one who recognizes the potential his mate has and helps her develop it. He somehow senses that as she gets a greater sense of self-worth, she has more love to give him. He is not threatened by her talents; he encourages them.

If the woman in your life wants to go back to school to complete her education or perhaps get an advanced degree, do everything in your power to convince her that she is capable of doing it. If she wants to get a job, change jobs, or be considered for a promotion, tell her you are behind her one hundred percent. Alleviate her anxieties about the home front by developing a plan in which you will spend more time helping with the kids and the chores.

Anne is one of those women who will be eternally grateful to her husband for all his encouragement. "I was a full-time housewife most of our married life," she began. "When the kids finally went off to college, I was faced with free time and nothing to do that couldn't be done in a few hours. When I told Charlie I wanted to get a job, he said that was a great idea. He even went shopping with me to buy a new outfit, complete with shoes and handbag, to wear on my interviews.

"I began as a temporary secretary in a large construction firm. Every night, Charlie asked me all about my day and seemed so interested in what I had to say. Later, as my job became more demanding and I got a promotion, my wonderful husband suggested we go out to dinner three times a week because he knew how exhausted I was. He began helping me around the house with the wash, cooking dinner, and vacuuming. I felt like we were really a team. His confidence in me helped me feel confident about myself. I'm the envy of all my friends, having a husband like Charlie."

When I finally felt brave enough to put my first class together, it took a great deal of money to pay for leasing an office and advertising the classes. My husband encouraged me every step of the way. He took out a quite substantial loan to help cover all the expenses for the first year. At first I was losing money every month, but never once did he make me feel bad or guilty.

He'd always say, "Look, Ellen, the most important thing is that you enjoy what you're doing. If that's true, then the money will come." Never did he tell me that it was a terrible idea or that I wasn't going to make it. I honestly believe that had he said any of those things, I never would have begun, and even if I had begun, I probably would have quit.

## IN TOUCH WITH THE CHILD INSIDE

A man who is in touch with the child inside himself is the ultimate turn-on, because he possesses so many traits that women find attractive. He is playful, imaginative, and has the ability to dream. He is honest, curious, compassionate, and has the ability to enjoy the present.

Most of you at some point when you were reaching manhood heard your parents or teachers tell you, "Hurry up and grow up," or "Why don't you act your age?" or "Stop acting like a child." I actually heard a mother yell at her four-year-old son, who was giggling uncontrollably in a department store, "Stop acting so silly and act your age." I wanted to tell her, "Lady, he *is* acting his age!"

Most of you listened to your parents and teachers and followed their instructions, and in some cases, you've even exceeded their wildest expectations. You've exchanged your childish behavior for maturity. You are now a full-grown, full-time, mature adult male.

Others of you were lucky enough not to get that message, or else you got it and didn't listen to it. You are the ones who know the secret combination to unlocking a woman's heart.

## CHILDLIKE BEHAVIOR

Becoming a child again, being childlike, even if only from time to time, is one of the most endearing qualities a man can possess. Maybe, if you see as much value in it as I do, you will choose to bring it back again and make it part of your life. I know some of you had it shamed or punished out of you, so it's stuck way down deep inside, but with a little persistence, you can reclaim that vital part of you that would be so fulfilling to you and the woman you love.

*Children Are Playful*—In the movie *Big,* the character played by Tom Hanks has an adult body but the mind of a thirteen-year-old. A very contemporary, sophisticated woman is attracted to him. When she arrives at his apartment, he invites her to jump on his trampoline. She initially refuses, considering this to be a childish activity and certainly not something in which a woman of her stature would engage. He is very persistent and won't take no for an answer. She finally agrees, takes one jump, and says that's enough. He keeps encouraging her to jump some more, and before you know it, she is having the time of her life, jumping higher and higher. He was able to draw out the "little girl" in her and allowed her, once again, to become playful, a part of her she had forgotten existed. This is just one example of how refreshing playful behavior can be. In Chapter 7, "The Imaginative Lover," I'll give you many more examples.

*Children Are Imaginative*—A woman gets excited being with a man who has imagination. He can take her to faraway places without leaving home. He uses creative ways to make love to her, and most of all, he knows how to romance her. An imaginative man is never boring to be with.

*Children Are Dreamers*—Ask any child what he wants to be, do, or have, and you'll get the most incredible answers.

A man who still has a dream or a vision of what he still wants to experience and accomplish is a winner. Women are not attracted to aimless men who, night after night, sit in front of the TV watching other people's dreams come true. Just getting through the day or paying the bills is not a dream any woman would want to share.

*Children Are Honest*—Every child starts out completely honest. Ask, "Did you do that?" and children will tell you the truth. However, they soon discover that the truth can often lead to punishment. Children learn not to be honest, because when they are, they get into trouble. A woman has a very secure feeling being with a man who is always, without exception, honest with her. If she knows he will always be truthful, she trusts him with all her heart.

*Children Are Curious*—Their curiosity comes from a genuine interest in everything and everyone around them. A man who retains this ability is never bored. He always seeks new information that gives him new insight. His quest for knowledge never stops. His interest in other people means he'll always have friends and never experience loneliness. This kind of man never stagnates, because he is constantly growing.

*Children Are Compassionate*—A child can sense when you're unhappy and, with the most wonderful innocence, come over, sit on your lap, and just hug you. When my son was very young, and he'd see me feeling a little down, he'd just come up to me and say, "Mommy, I love you." Somehow that always did the trick.

Author and lecturer Leo Buscaglia once talked about a contest he was asked to judge. The purpose of the contest was to find the most caring child. The winner was a four-year-old child whose next-door neighbor was an elderly gentleman who had recently lost his wife. Upon seeing the man cry, the little boy went into the old gentleman's yard, climbed onto his lap, and just sat there. When his mother asked him what he had said to the neighbor, the little boy said, "Nothing, I just helped him cry." An invaluable man is one who can put his arms around his mate and help her cry, or just say, "I love you, sweetheart."

*Children Know How to Enjoy the Present*—John Lennon once wrote, "Life is what happens to you while you're busy making other plans." Many men do not know how to enjoy the present. They are either living in the past or have anxiety about the future. Another quote I've used many times is "Yesterday is a canceled check, tomorrow is a promissory note, today is cash in the bank." Have you ever watched a child playing? Children are not concerned with time. They don't care about ten minutes ago or ten minutes from now. Their total concentration and enjoyment centers around each moment. What if you could now do the same? What if you could enjoy each moment of your life as it happens, instead of living so many of your days anxiously awaiting some future event? Take inventory of everything you possess right now and delight in it. You'll be surprised at just how much you do have.

I remember one woman who was married to a construction foreman. At work he was known as "Stormin' Norman," but at home her pet name for him was "Studmuffin."

I suspect that every woman wants a studmuffin to live with. Two of my favorite public personalities who are definitely studmuffins are Bill Cosby and Phil Donahue. Both men allow the "little boy" to come out and play. Donahue, with his wide-eyed mannerisms and childlike curiosity, and Cosby, with his voice and facial expressions, have captured the hearts of women everywhere. Telly Savalas, playing Kojak, has also earned the right to be inducted into the Studmuffin Hall of Fame. Here he is, a rough-and-tough detective who sucks on a lollipop. Of course Kojak is only a fictitious character, but he lets you know that under that lion's roar is a pussycat. These men leave no doubt that although they can be playful, they are also men who possess great strength of character.

For some of you, that "little boy" is just waiting for permission to come out. For others, he's hiding a little deeper, but call on him anyway. Give him permission to call on the "little girl" inside that woman beside you.

## ACTION ASSIGNMENT #5

1. Look at the list of turn-offs and turn-ons and decide which traits you need to work on.
2. Check out one book on personal growth from the library.
3. Make an attempt to be more playful this week.
4. If she's going through a stressful period, put your arms around her and tell her to lean on you. If you are going through some tough times, lean on her.
5. If she asks your opinion, give it, but remember that it's only an opinion. You're not laying down a law.

6. If a decision has to be made, make sure you ask her opinion.
7. If you've been extremely jealous, tell her how sorry you are and how you are going to work on trusting her more.
8. Take one day off from work this week just to stop and smell the flowers, feel the sunshine, and enjoy the fresh air. Instead of a day off due to illness make it a day for pleasure.
9. Sit down one evening and ask her if she has anything she wants to do or complete. Encourage her, give her confidence, and tell her you'll help any way you can.

Dear Ellen,

I thought romance was only possible in novels and movies, but my level-headed, logical, practical husband has turned into a regular Don Juan. He has arranged romantic weekend getaways, moonlight walks on the beach, picnics in the park, and afternoon rendezvous. I, on the other hand, have become a wild, passionate woman. Thanks for bringing out a whole new dimension in our lives.

Love,
Millie

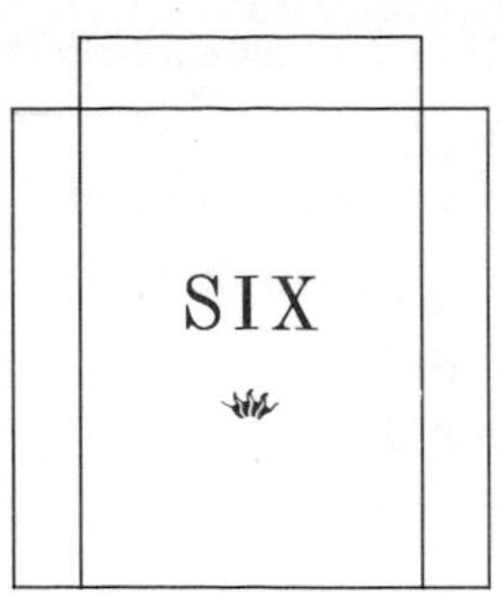

# SIX

## *Romance Me*

### IT'S YOUR TURN

Women have always been told in every book that has been written on the subject:

> Wear sexy outfits, scanty lingerie, garter belts and stockings, and any other outfit that is visually appealing to turn your man on.
>
> Don't walk around in curlers and rollers with cold cream on your face. Make sure your hair is beautifully styled and makeup applied properly so that you look as attractive as possible. After all, you don't want him to find someone he works with more attractive.
>
> Have the house in order so that he can come home to a haven of peace and tranquility.
>
> Make sure you cook his favorite foods, because the way to a man's heart is through his stomach.

She's told that if she doesn't do these things, he'll lose interest and have an affair with someone else. I happen to agree with all of this and based *Light His Fire,* my book for women, on these principles.

The only problem with these instructions is that she won't want to do any of them unless she gets something more than the promise that you won't go out and make love to another woman. It's not a fair deal.

We're now in the nineties, and the fifties woman is gone. Forty years ago, women did everything to please their men with no expectations in return. They had no identity of their own, so their lives were completely in the hands of their husbands.

Today's woman has a mind of her own, as well as a career of her own. She has options and choices.

- No longer does she have to be married to have sex.
- No longer does she have to stay married because it's difficult to get a divorce.
- No longer does society frown upon a divorced woman.
- No longer does she have to be married to have a child.
- No longer does she have to remain in a marriage because she can't earn a living.
- No longer does she have to stay married for the sake of her children.

Today's woman will remain married or loyal to one man only if she feels her needs are being fulfilled. Do you know the saying, "What's good for the goose is good for the gander"? I've always said to women, "If you don't have a love affair with your man, someone else will." On the other hand, a woman today can say, "If you don't have a love affair with me, then another man will!" Staying with you has to be a "want to" for her, because she no longer "has to." For her to remain loyal and want to spend the rest of her life with you, you must learn what she's looking for in a man, what she desires in a relationship, and what it takes to fulfill her needs. Otherwise, you may find yourself alone.

## SO YOU'RE NOT PERFECT

When I teach the men in my classes what a woman is looking for in a man to keep her hopelessly and passionately in love with them, many times they respond with the following:

- I'm not the sensitive type.
- I can't communicate with women.
- I'm not comfortable with myself.
- I'm not a touchy-feely person.
- I find it hard to open up.
- I'm very reserved.
- I'm not creative or imaginative.
- I worry too much about the future to enjoy the present.
- I'm not a fun guy.
- I'm never satisfied with anything.

There are many reasons why men are not romantic. Over the past nine years, several men in my classes have admitted to not having one romantic bone in their bodies.

Carl said, "I never saw my parents do anything but argue. They never kissed, at least not in front of me, or showed any affection of any kind. The truth is, I just don't know what to do."

For Carl and countless other men who had no role models, being open and caring is a completely foreign feeling. If you didn't grow up seeing your father do romantic things for your mother, it's probably difficult for you to do these things for your mate.

For Martin, it was the fear of rejection. He shared, "I'm always scared that I'll make a fool of myself. What if I do something romantic, and she winds up laughing at me? I don't want her to think I'm corny or stupid."

Fear of rejection is another common reason for not developing your romantic side. Everyone wants acceptance. But this is more than acceptance. This is wanting another person to find you desirable and sexy. She might laugh the first time you leave her a mushy note or a silly little gift, but if you do it with all your heart, that note or that little gift will become a treasure to her. So take a chance, and you'll be surprised how good you can make both of you feel.

Andy attributes his lack of romance to laziness. "It's just too much work. I'd rather sit back and have it done to me." For Andy, the thought of putting time and effort into showing a woman how much he cares is just too exhausting. Andy feels he has to work at his job. Why work at a relationship? He doesn't realize that just as he'll receive the payoff from his efforts at work, so, too, will he receive a payoff at home. The payoff will be a happy, loving, supportive, passionate woman instead of the depressed, angry, cold, bitter, unsupportive woman that he now has.

The list goes on and on as to why men think it's impossible to add a dimension to their lives that they weren't born with. So you have a choice. You can be like Carl, Martin, and Andy, who all seem to have valid reasons for not being romantic and will eventually wind up by themselves, or you can decide to educate yourself as much as possible by reading books or going to a psychologist for help to learn how to change your reaction to women. I'm not asking you to change your basic core as a person, only the way you treat another human being—mostly the woman in your life. Let's see how easy this is to do.

Nobody is walking around this earth perfect. People just aren't born with the characteristics necessary to live full, productive lives without first experiencing pain, hurt, and disappointment. They say experience is the best teacher. I agree. Constant feedback from other people, and events in our lives over which we have no control, force us to move forward and grow. Life is constant movement, and new information often brings new behavior.

## BIOLOGY VERSUS PSYCHOLOGY

If a couple has a great sex life, I know each partner has been a wonderful teacher, and each has learned a valuable lesson. In Chapter 1, I said that opposites attract, that we each have something to learn from our mate, that we each have something to teach them.

## MEN ARE BIOLOGICAL. WOMEN ARE PSYCHOLOGICAL.

It's usually a man who ultimately teaches a woman that her body is beautiful and something to be proud of and enjoy. He also teaches her to become more physical, to enjoy sex, to relax and have fun. This is so natural for a man, because most of his life he reacts in a physical way. A man gets sexually aroused by looking at magazines, X-rated movies, or long legs. His response is immediate, and his reactions tend to be physical.

If a man is a truly great lover, he has been taught tenderness, understanding, appreciation, sensitivity, and patience. For a woman, sex is not an immediate reaction. It's usually a decision she makes mentally, not physically, when she is in the mood for sex. Most women have to give themselves permission to get aroused sexually. For a woman, if there is not a feeling of closeness, caring, and understanding, she will not respond in the bedroom. Her mind is in control of her body.

Sally did a good job of summing up many women's feelings when she told the class, "All Jerry ever wanted was sex. He never talked or even held me. In fact, he stopped kissing, too. When I turned off to making love, he called me frigid. Then he took 'Light Her Fire' and became a tender, loving, and warm man instead of a mechanical robot. Now I'm turned on again. I just can't separate sex from our relationship. They are the same thing to me."

When a man and woman have been together for many years, there's a give and take that's apparent when they speak about how each has helped the other grow by meeting the other's needs.

Margaret said that she was terribly shy and embarrassed about her body until Ruben came into her life. She said, "He kept saying over and over how beautiful I was. He'd bring home those sexy nightgowns, which took all of my courage to put on, but then the look on his face and the smile on his lips would put me at ease. He'd spend hours cuddling, stroking, and massaging me, all the while reinforcing how much I meant to him. After a while, I couldn't help but respond. Now I feel so much better about my body. I actually enjoy wearing different sexy outfits to excite him."

## EMOTIONAL VERSUS PHYSICAL

If a woman's emotional needs are not met, she can't respond to you physically. I also know it's hard for you to respond emotionally to her unless your physical needs have been met. We are so different, and yet someone has to take that first step. If you will learn how a woman wants to be loved, then she'll respond in a way you never dreamed possible.

I polled a group of men and women and asked them, "What is the most pleasurable time you spend with the woman or man you love?"

Most of the men responded, "When we are making love."

However, the women responded in a completely different way. Not one said, "Having sex." Their list consisted of hugging, touching, kissing, and talking. Not the sex act.

The most powerful knowledge you can have about how to turn a woman on is to know that *a woman is receptive to making love only when her emotional needs have been met.*

## SEX IS GIVING

Sex for her is kindness, gentleness, devotion, commitment, caring, patience, and compliments. It starts in the morning with whether you said "I love you" before you left. It's telling her how much she means to you. It's going shopping with her. It's helping her with the chores. It's noticing that she has a new dress or hairdo. It's asking her to dinner. It's whether you phoned to say you'll be late. It's bringing home a card or a gift. Real romance for a woman is letting her know she's special, appreciated, and loved. It's you spending time reaching out to her in a very giving way.

This is very different from what most men are used to. Listen in on any locker-room talk in a high school, and boys will ask each other, "Did you get anything last night?" "Did you score?" "Did you conquer her?" These are not tender, loving questions. They are very selfish, immature questions, yet men of all ages operate on this level, consciously and unconsciously, until either catastrophe or enlightenment comes.

So give her little things—your attention, your caring, your kindness—and you will receive more from her than you ever hoped for. Unlike most men, a woman will not be in the mood to make love just because you are there. She'll be in the mood because you are nice to her.

## ATTENTION TO NEEDS

If you were a salesman trying to sell your product to a particular company, the first thing you would do is find out what that company's needs are. If the company you were calling on cared mostly about progressive thinking, about being on the leading edge of technology, about being an innovator in their field, and price was not their main concern, you'd lose the sale if you tried to sell your product on the basis of price competitiveness. Why? Because you didn't pay attention to what they were saying. You didn't fulfill their needs. On the other hand, another company interested only in price would not buy from you if you emphasized that your product would help build their image.

A woman, like a company, will tell you her needs. You just have to listen. And you can't make a value judgment that says, "The way you want to be loved is wrong. My way is better."

If a woman says, "I need to know you love me," a man may respond with, "I'm working my tail off to provide a living. Isn't that enough?" This is *not* listening. It is quite possible that she sees your job as an obligation you have only to yourself, not a fulfillment of her emotional needs.

Dominic shared with the class, "I was the manager of the customer complaint department of a large corporation. All day long I listened to people's problems and complaints. I certainly wasn't in the mood to come home and hear my wife do the same thing. When she'd start telling me about the problems she was having with our two teen-age sons, I'd get annoyed with her and say, 'Look, all day long I'm solving problems; I'm not about to spend my evenings doing the same. All I want is peace and quiet. I don't think that's too much to ask.' That usually stopped her cold. The only problem was that later, when I wanted to make love to her, she remained cold. After the first few classes, I really started to think about what I was doing to her. I was giving myself to other people I didn't even know, but not to my wife. All she was asking for was time to talk about her frustrations and anxieties. She needed some help, and she wanted a little guidance from me. Once I started listening and being there for her, you can bet she was there for me later in the evening."

Charles, too, received some new insight as to why Tanya was having trouble responding to him. "The truth is," he said, "I sometimes paid more attention to other women and gave them more compliments than I did my wife. It didn't matter whether it was a waitress serving us or a friend coming over to the house. I always said something to make them feel good. When Tanya told me she needed to know that I was still attracted to her, I countered with, 'Well, you're the one I live with, and I don't fool around, do I?' 'No,' she said, but she still couldn't help feeling jealous and cheated. She accused me of having no compliments left, since I had so generously dished them out to everyone but her. As a result of the classes, I finally realized that she, too, needed to hear how pretty, sexy, smart, and wonderful I thought she was. All I had been giving her was the assurance that I was being faithful. It just wasn't enough."

Daryl didn't think that gifts were necessary to show you love someone. Every time Patricia got upset at not receiving something for her birthday or anniversary, Daryl responded with, "You have everything a person could want. You have a beautiful home, a nice car, and as far as I can see, you are well dressed. Why do you make these stupid demands for gifts? You're never satisfied with what you have. You always want more."

Ironically, Daryl felt the same way about their sex life. It was never enough. He always wanted more. But he will never get more, because he doesn't know how to respond to Patricia's needs outside the bedroom.

If she asks for flowers, don't give her a kitchen utensil. If she asks you to call her during the day, don't give her a story about how you're too busy trying to make a living for her. Your attention, your obvious caring, is more important to her than any amount of money you might bring home. Listen to what she is saying. A woman will tell you constantly what she needs in order to respond to you sexually.

For a woman, sex is not the act of intercourse. The real foreplay takes place sometimes hours before the sexual act. Perhaps a better word for this is forethought. Your thoughtfulness can be the ultimate turn-on for her.

## HE'S VISUAL—SHE'S VERBAL

A man gets excited looking at pictures of women in alluring outfits, negligees, erotic poses, etc. Sometimes just a woman with long legs or large breasts will be enough to arouse him. That's why in my first book, *Light His Fire,* I gave women many ideas that emphasized pleasing men visually.

A woman, however, gets more excited by words. She loves reading romance novels, while he enjoys reading *Playboy.* Not too many men I know buy Harlequin novels. In fact, if I happen to be reading a romantic book, my husband will lean over my shoulder and ask, "Where are the good parts?" I think you know what he's referring to.

A man who is watching an X-rated film could care less

about the plot. Most women watching the same film might say, "Why can't they make it a good story with intelligent dialogue?"

"I remember concentrating so hard on the story," Lynne volunteered. "Finally, I told my husband I didn't get it. He looked at me in disbelief and said, 'There's nothing to get!' "

Many men love movies like *Rambo* and *The Terminator* because they can see action; they aren't looking for meaningful dialogue. But let a woman see *An Officer and a Gentleman,* where the hero and heroine have captured her heart, then watch her get excited. Meaningful dialogue and warmth prior to lovemaking is what really turns a woman on.

Remember, *a man reacts sexually to what he sees, but a woman reacts sexually to what she hears or reads because they both involve words.*

## LOVE TO HAVE SEX, SEX TO HAVE LOVE

A man uses sex to have love. A woman needs love in order to have sex. That's why those three little words, "I am sorry," mean so much to a woman. If you've hurt her in some way by being negligent or forgetful, either begin with saying you're sorry or writing a note that says, "Please forgive me."

She wants you to communicate with words, not your body. Many men have a tendency to use the sex act to show that they are sorry. They want to make love in order to make up with their mate. She needs you to make up with words first before she can make love. Then, when she feels close again, she can respond to you sexually. And remember, for her, it is not an immediate response. It takes her time to forgive.

Admitting that you made a mistake is not an act of weakness. It shows strength. A man who never takes responsibility or blame for anything he does or says is not someone a woman will feel loving toward.

Mac learned this the hard way. He said, "We were married less than six months, and I came home late without calling. When I finally got home around two A.M., I slipped into bed as quietly as I could and started kissing her. She turned to me and said, 'All you can think about is yourself.' I wasn't thinking about myself. I just wanted to make it up to her. Sex was the only way I knew to reach out and say I was sorry. I realize now that she needed to hear it. What I should have done was say, 'Honey, I'm so sorry. I got so wrapped up in Vincent's problems that we went for a drink, and the next thing I knew, it was one o'clock. Please forgive me. I promise it won't happen again. You know I love you and would never do anything to hurt you. Tomorrow, let's go out for breakfast and talk about it.' I know if I had done that, I could have avoided the cold-shoulder treatment she gave me for three days."

## LOOKING FORWARD TO SOMETHING

Women are future oriented. They have a difficult time concentrating on the here and now. When a woman first falls in love, she begins to think, "What kind of husband will he be?" or "He'll make a great father." She loves to plan ahead.

Women are the ones who make early preparations for the holiday months. They buy presents early, in most cases at least a few weeks ahead, trying to avoid the last-minute rush. This year, I deliberately went to a major shopping mall in my area after three o'clock on December 24, Christmas Eve. As I looked around, I found the stores filled with men. A saleslady came up to me and said, "What are you doing here so close to Christmas? Usually it's a frantic boyfriend looking for anything that's within his price range." We both laughed, and yet there was so much truth in her comment.

*A woman has to have something to look forward to.* Keeping in mind the importance a woman puts on the future, you have to come up with something special that will ensure her future happiness. That's why women love dates. It gives us something to look forward to. It's an acknowledgment from you to her. There are many reasons for that acknowledgment. The following are just a few examples.

> "I know you've been through a great deal lately, and I want to show you how much I appreciate you."
> "I know I've been neglecting you, and I want to make it up to you."
> "I've been concentrating on me, and it's time to concentrate on us."
> "You've been working so hard lately, you deserve some time out for fun."

Gil couldn't wait to tell the class how he put this information to work immediately. He is a hunter, and prior to hunting season, which was coming up shortly, his life always became a nightmare. Rose, his wife, usually did everything she could to make him feel guilty for leaving her and the children so he could spend time with the "boys." She would complain continuously about how she'd have all the responsibility while he had all the fun.

This year, Gil took Rose in his arms and said, "Honey, you know how much hunting means to me, and I'm so thankful for having a wife that takes care of everything while I'm gone. I know it's hard on you, so let's make a deal. When I get back, I'll make the arrangements, and we'll go away the following weekend, just the two of us."

He said Rose felt his forehead to see if he had a fever. When he assured her that he was not delirious, just more aware of what she needed, she began to melt. "She's been singing around the house ever since and even went shopping for some extra things I needed for the trip. She also told me she'd give me a night to remember when I left and a night to look forward to on my return. I can't believe it's the same woman."

Gordon, who frequently goes away on business, always expected a home-cooked meal when he got back because he ate out on the road so much. He never understood why his wife was so upset when he left but not that eager when he returned. He began to see that although he was happy with his job and the future, Vicki was always exhausted when he returned from his trips. All this changed. Gordon made a pact with Vicki. Whenever he returned from a trip, they would go out to eat that first night. It would be their date night. The relief he saw in his wife's face was instantaneous. Later he reported that now his returns were very romantic, and instead of concentrating on cooking and cleaning, Vicki had the energy to concentrate on creative lovemaking.

Alan, like so many other men, loves watching football on Monday nights. Prior to his taking my class, which was right in the middle of football season (luckily, the class met on Tuesday nights), he was watching less and less TV at home. Married for only five years, the last two had been going from bad to worse.

Gina would start nagging on Friday evening, because she knew that Sunday and Monday were Alan's days to tune her out and tune football in. As soon as they both got home from work, she'd either start in with a list of things she expected him to accomplish over the weekend or complain about the things he hadn't done. By Sunday, the arguments would be going full blast, causing him to storm out of the house. He'd either wind up at a neighbor's house or a local pizza parlor with a wide-screen TV.

Eager to try anything, he suggested to Gina that they call a truce. If she would let him relax on Sunday during the day and on Monday nights, he'd take her to dinner and a movie of her choice on Wednesday evenings. The last I heard, Alan is not only back in his own home watching football, but Gina has popcorn and pretzels for him to enjoy, and they've been making some rather spectacular tackles in the bedroom.

## RECONNECT AND BE FREE

There is absolutely nothing wrong with having separate careers or different interests or spending time in the pursuit of individual endeavors as long as you remember to reconnect when you haven't been with each other for any length of time. The reconnection should always be a special event. You've been focusing on other things, and now it's time to focus on each other. If you don't, a woman is not going to respond to you sexually. The bonding, or reconnecting, is an absolute necessity for a woman to get turned on.

Marty stayed after class one night to complain about the lack of sexuality between him and his wife, Joan. "She used to be so wonderful in bed. She always responded to me. Now, nothing!" He was especially confused, he explained, since the previous Saturday night they'd gone to a friend's party and he thought they'd both had a good time. When they got home, he knew they could sleep late on Sunday because they had no commitments. When he began touching her, she immediately responded with, "You've got to be kidding! I'm exhausted, and I've got a headache. I'm not in the mood."

Marty reconsidered this great Saturday night. He recalled that Joan had been involved in conversation with the "girls," and he had been heavily engrossed in Fred's tales of remodeling his home. Not once during the evening did Joan and Marty connect. Joan needed that connection in order to respond sexually to Marty later.

Let's imagine a different scenario. Ten minutes into the party, Marty walked over to Joan and whispered in her ear, "You are the most beautiful woman here tonight." About a half hour later, he came over to her, put his arm around her waist, and asked if she needed a refill for her drink. Then, an hour and a half later, he walked over to her, grabbed her arm, and asked the girls if she could be excused for a few minutes because he needed to talk to her. When they had gone into one of the other rooms, he gave her a passionate kiss and said he couldn't wait to be alone with her, adding, "Just thinking about making love to you takes my breath away!" When they left the party, he held her hand, and he stopped to give her another kiss before they got into the car.

Had Marty done all the things described in this alternate version, the ending of this story would be *Marty and Joan made passionate love.*

## TAKE ME AWAY FROM ALL THIS!

For most women, home represents work. She's always looking at the refrigerator that needs restocking, the floor that needs to be cleaned, the wash that has piled up, the dust that has accumulated, the dinner that needs to be prepared, the vacuuming that must be done, and possibly the children, who need to be bathed. This is not an environment that makes for a sex goddess.

On a routine basis, you have to take her away from all this. Your car can be your horse, and you'll be her knight in shining armor who rescues his princess from the daily stresses that come with running a household.

Women have a tendency to feel that they cannot leave the children because something might happen while they're away. They are usually filled with anxiety and guilt. She needs you to convince her that the only real tragedy that will happen if you don't go away once in a while is the loss of intimacy you'll both experience. You must recapture your focus on each other. It's money well spent when you see the results a mini-getaway achieves. Most couples wouldn't think of getting married without having a honeymoon. Think of these vacations as mini-moons. This is the time when you can get your lover back. The inhibitions that exist at home because of lack of privacy due to children, friends that drop by, or just the phone ringing don't exist when you are away. Help her find a suitable baby-sitter, if children are involved, so she feels more comfortable. Plan these mini-moons well in advance so you can make all the arrangements necessary for a smooth getaway.

My husband and I have a long-standing agreement. Whenever either of us has to travel on business, the very next available weekend is ours to plan an overnight stay at a nearby hotel. The Irvine Hilton and Towers Hotel is only fifteen minutes from our house, but they have a "Bounce Back Weekend" that they advertise as a stress reliever. Boy, is that the truth! There is usually so much tension in any home where two people have not spent enough time with each other that you can cut it with a knife. The hotel also has a wise motto that says, "Why drive, when you can relax in your own backyard?" Most people think they have to go to a distant place to unwind. Sometimes, a perfect getaway is right nearby. Check the local hotels in your own area for their weekend specials.

Remember, you will have to sacrifice time, money, and effort, but I'd rather see energy spent on wonderful future memories than time, money, and effort spent in a marriage counselor's office.

If you don't get away together every now and again, just to be alone together, you will become strangers. You'll lose touch with each other, and the price you'll pay for that is enormous. And don't worry about the children. The best gift you could ever give your children is a loving relationship with your wife.

If you don't have children, and your careers are so hectic they infringe on any personal time away together, when you do take that much-needed break, you'll have much more energy when you go back to work. Time spent concentrating exclusively on each other has an energizing effect. You'll have more stamina and think more clearly when you remove yourself from the daily stresses we all have to go through. But best of all, you'll be back in touch with the most important person in your life.

## GROOMING HABITS

So many women have voiced this complaint in over nine years of classes that I feel I must bring it up. If you are about to spend any length of time with your mate, whether it is going on a date or spending the weekend at home with her, you need to pay attention to grooming habits.

Most women want to feel they are worth going to some trouble for. When you make that extra effort in preparation for spending time with your mate, she takes that as proving your love once again. When you first dated, you got ready for the evening. You took pains to make sure that you looked as good as you could for her. Being presentable for her was an important part of the courtship, and courtship makes a woman feel as if she's the most important person in your life. Even now, she'll accept nothing less than that and deserves the same thoughtfulness throughout your life together.

If you live alone, there's no one else to consider or prepare for, but once you have a living arrangement with a woman, there is more than just yourself to consider. On your first date with this wonderful woman, would you have dared not showering, shaving, brushing your teeth, putting on cologne, and wearing presentable clothes? Not on your life! I know you do this every day when getting ready for work.

What message does the most important person in your life get when she sees you doing these things every day for your job, and all she gets is a tired, sweaty, odorous body at the end of the day? The message is, "He goes to all this trouble for strangers and people he will never see again, but not for me." It comes down to, "Others are worth his time and effort, and I'm not."

Floyd admitted to being guilty in this area. "You know, it's so true what Ellen is saying. All week long I get dressed up to go to my office, so on weekends I put on an old worn-out pair of jeans and my ripped T-shirt. I don't feel like shaving, because I've done that every morning for five days. Janet always pushes me away when I try to kiss her, telling me my face feels like sandpaper. The only time I turn her on is when I'm walking out the door to go to work in the morning."

Why is it that we treat perfect strangers with such consideration and the people we love the most with a "the-heck-with-you" attitude? If you've been guilty, start with one small step. Pick any one day and do what you did when you were dating. I'm going to assume that the reinforcement from your mate will be enough of an inducement to keep adding more days.

By the way, women are always encouraged to dress in sexy outfits. I suggest you invest in some silk pajamas, a lounging robe, and some sexy underwear. She'll be shocked and pleased that you have a special wardrobe for her, too.

## ROMANCE MEANS TOUCHING

For a woman, the lack of nonsexual touching is not only a loss of romance, but withholds from her the fulfillment of a basic human need, being physically close.

Most women complain that the only time a man will hold her or stroke her is when he wants sex or is having sex. Remember my basic belief that opposites attract? If you are not a toucher, you probably fell in love with a woman who loves to touch. But if every time she touches you, you immediately respond, "Let's go to bed," eventually she'll stop. Women need to be held and cuddled and stroked every single day, without exception. To her it's an end in itself. It doesn't have to lead anywhere.

Sidney explained that he had caused his wife to become distant this way. "When we first got married, Darlene loved touching me. She would massage my back, stroke my hair, rub my arm or leg, and she kissed me all the time. Every time she did, I'd get that gleam in my eye and tell her to get ready for some real love. I remember her looking so hurt, then angry, as she said, 'I thought just being together was real love.' Finally, five years later, I understand why she stopped touching me. She was afraid I would push her into the bedroom every single time she did it."

I think men in general don't do enough nonsexual touching. This has a great deal to do with our culture. Young American boys are taught early on that to touch another male affectionately is to subject themselves to ridicule. On the other hand, European men don't seem to have as much of a problem with this as American men. You always see men in Europe hugging and kissing each other. Russian men even kiss each other on the mouth to show affection.

For some reason, the only place male touching is acceptable in this country is in athletic competition. Football players are always patting each other on the rear end, and we think nothing of it. At the end of all competitive sports, the victors hug each other and usually display, publicly, a tremendous amount of affection for their teammates. Yet, outside of sports, men resort to a handshake, a pat on the back, a poke in the ribs, and a more reserved way of relating to each other in general.

I remember being at an airport waiting for my husband's arrival, and on an earlier flight a young boy of about twelve came off the plane running toward a man who appeared to be his father. The father, instead of hugging his son, stuck out his hand, stopping the young boy dead in his tracks. I overheard the father saying, "Boy, it's good to see you. It's been a long time," as he shook the young man's hand. I wanted to go over and take this man by the shoulders and say, "Why didn't you hug him?"

Many children, as well as women, are starving to be touched. They have "skin hunger." And believe it or not, you need to be touched as much as your mate does. So I would really like you to start a Touch Program outside the bedroom and begin to see the miraculous results it produces inside the bedroom.

Don't leave in the morning without giving her a hug. Even if you are both doing your own thing, every so often as you pass her, give her a hug, a kiss, or a pat so she feels connected to you. When you're watching TV together, hold her hand so she can feel your warmth. When you walk together, hold her hand or put your arm around her to let the world know you're together. Clinging to each other in bed gives her the reassurance that you love her and want to feel close to her. Begin the day that way and end the day in the same way.

Other loving actions are:

- Caressing her face
- Drying her tears
- Rubbing her back
- Massaging her feet
- Kissing her nose and eyes
- Massaging her neck

You might think that these things would just become part of a routine and have no meaning if you do them too often. You're wrong. Touching her just to touch her will always mean romance and love to a woman.

Have you ever seen a dog that doesn't want to be stroked daily? Somehow, we have become a dog- and cat-petting society. Many men who show absolutely no affection to their mates spend hours petting their animals. I want you to replace your animal with the woman in your life. It just might bring out the animal in her.

## AN INTIMATE WAY OF RELATING

Some men whisper terms of endearment and sweet nothings in their partner's ear while they are making love. I'd like to suggest that these terms of endearment and sweet nothings are also very important to a woman outside the bedroom. It's another way she feels very intimate with her mate. These pet names and phrases can only be reserved for someone you love. They don't apply to friends, neighbors, relatives, or co-workers, and that's what makes this kind of language so important to a woman.

You'd be shocked at the number of men who have never called their wives by anything but their first names. Gordon said, "Do you know, in all of our thirty-six years together, I've never called my wife anything but Evelyn. I've never thought of it before, but her good friends call her a variety of names which are abbreviated versions of her original name, like Eve, Evie, Lynn, or Lynnie. Even when we're making love, I call her Evelyn. I'm so reserved. Maybe I need to learn how to loosen up."

The following pet names are just suggestions that men have shared with me over the years. Some are so basic that many of you may wonder why I've included them, but I'll start out with the basic ones, then move to ones with a little more depth. Keep in mind that the men who use pet names or phrases have admitted to me privately that they not only use these when their mate is with them, but also on the phone and in writing notes to their special girl.

| | | |
|---|---|---|
| Honey | Poodle | Love Goddess |
| Baby | Dream Girl | Fireball |
| Babe | Candy Girl | My Enchantress |

Sweetheart
Darling
My Love
Hun
Sugar
Sexy
Beautiful
Cookie
Brown Eyes
Blue Eyes
Cuddles
Munchkin
Golden Girl
Princess
Bunny Rabbit
Goldilocks
Sexy Legs
Lover Girl
Almond Joy
Lucious Lips
Sweet Cheeks
Cherry Cheeks
Mama Bear
Nuzzle Bod
Passion Flower
Light of My Life
Heart Throbber
Toast of the Town
My Treasure
Sweet Lips
Hot Lips
Queen of Hearts
China Doll
Crowning Glory
Little Cabbage

Now, I know some of you are thinking, "If I called my girlfriend or wife some of these names, she'd call for the men in the white coats to take me away and lock me up somewhere!" If you'll just take a chance and say it with sincerity and confidence, not in a joking manner, she may find it strange or shocking at first, but it's a behavior she'll have fun with and enjoy getting used to.

If you've never done anything like this before, then try an easy one first and gradually add some new ones.

## FIFTY-ONE WAYS TO KEEP HER FIRE LIT

There is no reason for any couple to have a boring life together. Remember, boredom is repetition and predictability. So, to prevent boredom from happening to you, I am including fifty-one romantic ideas that you can use to impress, excite, and arouse the woman in your life. Remember, some of these ideas may not seem romantic to you, but I can assure you that they will be to a woman.

For a woman, romance is making her feel special. You don't do this for your colleagues, friends, or relatives. You do this just for her.

1. **Display Her**—Tell her you'd love to have a recent photograph of her to carry in your wallet or display at work. Make an appointment with a photographer for her to have a sitting for a portrait. If money is a problem, get out your own camera. Have her change into several outfits as you click away. Later, really concentrate on which proofs you like the most. The message this sends to a woman is, "He wants everyone to see that I'm his mate. He must think I am pretty; otherwise he wouldn't do this."
2. **Sing to Her**—Make an "I love you" call from the office. Call her and tell her you were just thinking about her and how much she means to you and you just wanted to say, "I love you." If you have a good voice, you can sing a few bars of Stevie Wonder's song, "I Just Called to Say I Love You." Go ahead and sing it even if you don't have a good voice!
3. **Go for Supermarket Specials**—Go to the supermarket and buy some of her favorite magazines, candy bars, and flowers. Bring them home and tell her she deserves to be showered with gifts because she's special, and you want her to relax in bed tonight eating her favorite candy and reading her magazines. Arrange the flowers by her bed.
4. **Circle the Dates**—Buy a calendar and circle any four days during the year you choose. Tell her that on

these dates you have a special night with her planned. Buy tickets to a concert or a play, or any other event you don't attend regularly. Include an overnight stay, if possible, at a local hotel. Make up a list of items she'll need to bring with her if you plan the hotel stay—or better yet, have an overnight bag already packed without her knowing it. Just circle dates far enough in advance so that you can put your thinking cap on and make more than adequate preparations. Remember, a woman loves for you to be in charge, preparing the evening just for the two of you. Anticipation is half the fun.

5. **Give Her a Rest**—If you have small children, shock her on Friday night with a single rose and a note on her pillow that says, "This note invites you to sleep in as long as you want tomorrow morning, because you deserve it! Your loving husband will take care of the children. When you do get up, plan to spend a few hours all to yourself. Go shopping and enjoy!" Watch out for that rested woman when she gets hold of you!
6. **Be the Groom Who Carries the Bride**—The next time you come to the front door together, sweep her off her feet and hold her in your arms as you carry her over the threshold. When she starts giggling and asking what you are doing, tell her you are carrying your lovely bride, whom you adore more now than the day you got married, over the threshold. Be very specific as you carry her. Look into her eyes and say, "I adore you more now than when we first got married!" Inside that practical, logical man there is a Casanova! You can do it!

7. A CARD EACH DAY YOU'RE AWAY—If you're going on a business trip, plan ahead. Buy enough cards (or write notes) so that each day you are away, you can call her and tell her to look for a card that you have hidden somewhere in your home prior to your departure. End each conversation with, "Honey, I love you. Now go to my middle dresser drawer and find a note for you." The next day she can look for a note in her sewing box, or tucked in the phone book, or clipped to a hanger in a closet. Just use your imagination.
8. CREATE A CEREAL HIDEAWAY—Buy a very sexy nightgown, wrap it in a small package, and hide it in a cereal box or any other place she'd least expect to find such an item.
9. PUT STICK-ON NOTES EVERYWHERE—Buy stick-on notes and put them all over the house. Write messages such as *I love you; You are beautiful; You mean the world to me; Our children are lucky to have a mom like you; I'm so lucky to have such a wonderful wife; You've got beautiful eyes.* You can even stick one on the toilet tissue roll in the bathroom!
10. SAY IT WITH SATIN—Wait until a department store is having a white sale and buy satin sheets. You'll need a bottom sheet, a top sheet, and pillow cases, and you'll need to know whether you have a king, queen, or full-size bed. Secretly put them on the bed. If you can, drape a silky nightgown across her pillow, and enjoy her response when she climbs into bed that evening.
11. TAKE THE DAY OFF—Take a day off from work; this really proves that you love her. Tell her you are hers all day to do whatever she wants. That may include

catching up on some chores, just taking a walk, or going shopping. Make the decision ahead of time that this is a lesson in giving, not receiving. The key is to be in a great mood for her all day. The message she gets is this: *You mean more to me than my work. I want to prove my love to you.*

12. **Make a Public Display**—If you are together in public, hold her hand, give her a kiss, put your arm around her shoulder. Show the world you enjoy being close to her.
13. **Give Her a Bubble Bath**—Buy some bubble bath and in the evening prepare a hot bath for her. Put some candles in the bathroom and turn off the lights. Bring in a portable radio and find some soft music. Tell her that you want her to relax, then take her hand and lead her to the bathroom. After her bath, provide her with a soothing massage.
14. **Set a Lunch Date**—Schedule a lunch date with her. The idea that you are taking time out from your busy day to have lunch with her will make her feel special. If you tell her you are putting it down in your appointment calendar, it will make her feel even more important.
15. **Take Her First Class**—Rent a limousine for the evening and tell her you're going first class because she is first class!
16. **Send Her on a "Present" Hunt**—Send her on a hunt for a present. Begin with note #1 on her pillow in the morning. Tell her something you like about her in the note and send her at an appointed time to note #2, and so on. End up at your mailbox and have a

present in it. This takes a bit of imagination, but I know you are capable of developing the creative side you have.

17. **Send Her on a "Love" Hunt**—A variation of the present hunt with notes, this is a more costly game. Leave a note and send her to a lingerie store in your area. Once there, she has to ask for a specific person and identify herself. That person will have a gift (picked out by you the day before) waiting for her and a note sending her to the neighborhood liquor store. There, she is handed a bottle of wine or champagne and a note sending her to a record store. There, you have a very romantic tape waiting for her and a note sending her to the florist. The florist should have a single long-stemmed rose waiting, along with a final note sending her to a restaurant you think she'd enjoy. Be waiting at the restaurant for her and make the rest of the evening something to remember.
18. **Send a No-occasion Gift**—A "no-occasion" gift or flowers sent to her office lets her co-workers know how much she is loved. To a woman this spells romance. When women are asked whether they prefer having flowers delivered or having them brought home by their husbands or boyfriends, most vote for deliveries.
19. **Buy Her a Dress**—Tell her that the next Saturday you are hers for the entire day, that you want to go shopping with her and buy her a new dress. Don't forget to add, "Because you deserve it!" Your whole week will be pleasant because of her anticipation.
20. **Make Love with Roses**—Go to the florist and buy

some long-stemmed roses. Be sure to have the thorns removed. While she's getting ready for bed, arrange them on the sheets and tell her you've always wanted to make love to her in a bed of roses. You can do a variation of this by using just the rose petals in bed and using the same explanation.

You can also surprise her by putting rose petals or other fragrant flowers in her bath. I know it sounds corny to some of you, but she'll be describing what you said and did for the rest of your lives.

21. **Walk Under a Full Moon**—One evening when she least expects it, shut off the TV (make sure it is not in the middle of her program) and tell her you would rather just be with her. Take a nice long walk and hold hands. Make a wish on a star and give her a nice long kiss.

    For an even more dramatic effect, look up in a farmer's almanac (which is published yearly in the fall for the next year) when the moon will be full for each month of that year. Put those dates down in your calendar and take a walk on those nights.

22. **Relive Your Teen Years**—Take her to a drive-in movie. Relive your teen years and fog up the windows.

23. **Compliment Her**—Next time you're with another couple, compliment your mate in front of them. She may act embarrassed, but secretly she'll love it. Remember, a compliment has three times the impact when it is said in front of someone else.

24. **Write a Love Letter**—Write her a love letter. Buy some extra-special stationery. Many stationery stores have special sheets that you can buy by the piece. Tell

her what she means to you and some of the wonderful memories you've shared together. These letters will be kept forever and someday may even be shared with your great-grandchildren.

25. **Read Poetry to Her**—Buy a beautiful book of poetry or check one out of the library and read her some of your favorite poems that you think apply to you and how you feel.
26. **Sing in the Rain**—The next time it rains, kick off your shoes, grab your sweetheart, and start singing "I'm Singing in the Rain." If you can, go to a music store to buy the lyrics and whip out the sheet music with a flourish so you can both sing in the rain.

    If you can't see yourselves doing this, then a nice variation is to sing in the shower together. Not only will you save water, but it is a lot of fun.
27. **Advertise Your Love**—Take out an advertisement in the personal section of a local newspaper. Tell her you love her and how important she is in your life. Add some of her most outstanding traits. Circle your ad and put it where she'll find it.
28. **Take a Class Together**—Take a class one night or day a week and learn something new together. It could be dancing lessons, bowling lessons, tennis lessons, golf lessons, a gourmet cooking class, a course on sailing, anything that involves the two of you. Most universities offer adult education classes that are interesting and fun. You may not be that enthusiastic initially, but just getting out together that one night will become enjoyable, and she'll love the fact that you want to do something solely with her.
29. **Plan a Cruise**—If you've never gone on a cruise

together, plan to try this fabulous way to take a vacation. Surprise her with different brochures from a travel agent and take a few weeks to decide where you want to go. I always recommend this kind of vacation because there are absolutely no decisions to be made. The biggest decision usually is which of the five entrees and six desserts to choose! You are waited on hand and foot. They have all kinds of activities and entertainment, and they usually go to exotic ports for shopping and sight-seeing. It's the ideal vacation. You'll come back more in love than when you left.

Remember, plan the trip far enough in advance so that she has something to look forward to for quite a while. In the meantime, you'll be living with a very content woman.

30. **Take a Train Trip**—Take her for an overnight trip on a train. Where you go is not nearly as important as being sure that you get a reservation in the sleeper car.
31. **Plan a Picnic**—Plan an old-fashioned picnic. Buy some wine, flowers, and sandwiches. Find a secluded spot and enjoy the warm sunshine. Bring along a radio for soft music, a book of poetry, and don't forget a blanket! You could also buy two kites and have fun being kids again.
32. **Sleep Under the Stars**—Sleeping under the stars is extremely romantic. You can do this in your own backyard. All you need is a sleeping bag or a blanket and some pillows.
33. **Dedicate a Trophy**—Buy her a trophy. Some women deserve a trophy even if they are not athletic. Have it engraved with her special achievements or

qualities, for example, to the best cook, the most attractive wife, most wonderful girlfriend. Be creative. The nice thing about trophy shops is that they carry silver-plated ice buckets, trays, and all kinds of other beautiful presents that you can personalize for that special someone.

34. **QUEEN FOR A DAY**—Make her "Queen for a Day." Buy a "diamond" tiara; costume rental shops usually have them. Tell her which day she will be queen, and explain that on that day, all her wishes will come true; tell her, "Your wish is my command." As long as it is in your power, you will grant her anything. Tell her to close her eyes as you put the tiara on her head and crown her your very own Queen for a Day.
35. **BREAKFAST IN BED**—Bring her breakfast in bed. Most department stores sell a breakfast tray of some sort. This is a great investment, as it can be used for both of you over the years. Buy a single rose and vase to hold it. Make her breakfast and surprise her with food and a beautiful flower. What a way to have her start the day!
36. **BUY A MUSIC BOX**—Buy her a music box that plays a romantic tune. While you wind it up, give her a kiss and tell her that every time she plays it, you want her to think of how much you love her.
37. **HERE'S LOOKING AT YOU**—Tape a note to her mirror that says, "Hello, beautiful, you are looking at the woman I love with all my heart. You take my breath away!"
38. **COOK A MEAL TOGETHER**—Plan to cook a meal together. Select some new recipe that both of you have

never tried. Bring the cookbook to bed and snuggle close as you decide which would be fun to try. Go shopping together for the ingredients and arrange the table setting together. Don't forget to kiss her frequently while cooking together. Use a French accent as you tell her you are "zee cooking chef."

39. **Relax Her**—Buy her the latest book by one of her favorite authors. After dinner, hand it to her and tell her to relax on the couch and read while you clean up. I can almost guarantee you'll get a reward later for being so wonderful.
40. **Ring Her Bell**—Buy a long-stemmed rose, and instead of coming in the house exhausted after a hard day of work, ring the doorbell. When she answers it, say, "Good evening, my sexy sweetheart. This is for you," and hand her the rose.
41. **Bring Home Dinner**—After you get to work, call her and tell her to have a great day and don't worry about dinner, because you'll be bringing it home. Music to her ears is you saying, "Honey, I'll take care of everything. Just have a wonderful day."
42. **Give a Grand Display**—Make a large banner on butcher paper that says I LOVE YOU, HAPPY BIRTHDAY, HAPPY ANNIVERSARY, or any other celebration. It could even be HAPPY FOUR MONTHS TOGETHER. Display it on the garage door—or better yet, on a freeway overpass—so everyone can see how much you care.
43. **Have a Romantic Toast**—Select the beach or woods. Ahead of time, take a card table there and cover it with a red-and-white checkered tablecloth. Set the table with some wineglasses and your favorite bottle of

wine. Add any edibles you'd like. Have a friend stand guard while you pick up your mate and bring her there for a romantic toast.

44. **Pick a Car Color**—This one can give a new meaning to travel. When the two of you are driving in a car, each of you must select a car color. Every time you see your car color, she has to give you a kiss. Every time she sees her car color, you have to give her a kiss. (Make sure you pick a common color!) At the end of the game, whoever has the most points (kisses) gets a wish granted. You can decide on the stakes at the beginning of your trip. You'll be shocked at how fast time flies when you're having fun.
45. **Service with a Kiss**—This one is a variation of the previous game. You have to be in a restaurant. Every time any waiter or waitress passes your table, you have to kiss each other. I don't know that you'll be all that hungry for food after you've played this one for a while.
46. **Pamper Her**—Give her a complete day of being pampered. Make arrangements for her to have a manicure, pedicure, facial, and hairstyling. Make sure it culminates with dinner for just the two of you. Comment on how radiant she looks. She'll be eager to tell you about the entire day's experiences.
47. **Be Artistic**—Give her a collage as a present. This can really bring out your creative ability. Get magazines and cut out pictures and sayings that have personal meaning for the two of you. Arrange them overlapping and at different angles. Glue your collage to posterboard and have it framed professionally. You

won't believe how fantastic it looks when it's done. The fun part will be sharing with her why you chose specific words and pictures.

48. **Give Her a Cassette**—Here's another easy way to be romantic: record your voice on a cassette tape. It can be a statement of how much you love her and why, followed by a poem you've found, and ending with a mix of songs you've selected that have special messages. Put a big bow on the cassette and leave it on her car seat with a note telling her how you'd really like her to listen to this while driving to work or leave it in a conspicuous place at home where she is sure to find it.
49. **Message in a Balloon**—Put messages in balloons about why she is so wonderful, for example, *You have a great sense of humor; You are a terrific kisser; I love your body.* Blow up the balloons and fill her car with them. Put a long needle on the windshield with a note saying that the only way she'll be able to get in her car is to pop each balloon and read the message.
50. **Give Her a Stuffed Animal**—There's not a woman alive who doesn't secretly want a beautiful, big, soft, stuffed animal. There are now so many to choose from, and when you add a personal note, it becomes irresistible. Here are some examples. A monkey with a note saying, "I'm ape over you—let's monkey around." A pig—"You drive me hog wild." A duck—"You can't duck my love for you." A gorilla—"I'm your prime mate." An elephant—"Let's kiss for the hellaphant." A cow—"I'm in the moo for love."

I know, corny, corny, corny, and yet not to a woman.

Her reaction will be, "Oh, how cute!" and she'll take it to bed with her, right along with you.

51. **Give Her a Party**—Throw her a Surprise-You-Are-Special party. Invite her friends and co-workers. Encourage them all to write something about why she's so wonderful. Plan a special toast to her. Yes, she will be embarrassed, but she will love every minute of it, and she will be the envy of every woman at your party.

A fantastic complement to any of the above ideas is a wonderful new game by Decipher Inc., which is based on all the principles I teach. It's called, "How to Host a Romantic Evening." The game enables you to have an evening of fun, romance, and intimacy. If you have a problem finding it in your local game store, send a self-addressed, stamped envelope for more information to:

LHF Enterprises
P.O. Box 1511
El Toro, CA 92630

There you have it, fifty-one ways to keep romance in your woman's life. Remember, *if a woman isn't fulfilled emotionally, she can't respond sexually.* Emotional fulfillment means you have gone out of your way, sacrificed, treated her with kindness, complimented her, made special time for her, and, most of all, you have made her feel as if she matters more to you than anyone else in this world. Good luck on your new romantic adventure!

## ACTION ASSIGNMENT #6

1. Plan a vacation together. It can be an overnight stay in a hotel, a weekend at a nearby resort, or a one-week holiday. Bring home brochures to look at, and plan it far in advance. Remember, she needs to have something to look forward to.
2. Once this weekend, get all dressed up as if you are going out. When she asks, "Where are you going?" take her in your arms and say, "Nowhere. I wanted to look special for you."
3. Begin a Touch Program and at least once each day physically touch her. Take her hand while you're walking, put your arm around her, kiss her gently, or make any other gesture that shows you enjoy being close to her.
4. Decide on a pet name for her and slip it in once this week. Be prepared for her to giggle.
5. Make a cuddle date with her. Send an invitation that says,

   **YOU ARE INVITED TO CUDDLE**

   | | |
   |---|---|
   | WITH WHOM: | ME |
   | WHEN: | FRIDAY EVENING AT 9:00 P.M. |
   | WHERE: | UNDER THE COVERS |

   Make some popcorn and bring in some Chinese food and snuggle and cuddle and talk all night long.
6. Read the list of "Fifty-one Ways" and decide which one you'd like to try out first. Then put your plan into action.

Dear Ellen,

I want to thank you for my new husband. When Gus enrolled in "Light Her Fire," we were both searching for the feelings we had somehow lost while we were busy raising five children. I believe we both settled for a routine, boring existence, and neither of us ever dreamed that there could be a whole new adventure waiting for us.

Gus has suddenly become the most imaginative, creative, exciting lover, even after thirty-two years of marriage. We have turned what had become at best a friendship back into a hot, torrid love affair. Gus has unleashed a part of himself that neither of us ever knew existed.

I find myself singing in the shower, at work, and even when I get stuck in heavy traffic. We both feel like teen-agers again.

Thank you from the bottom of my heart.

Forever grateful,

Lynnette

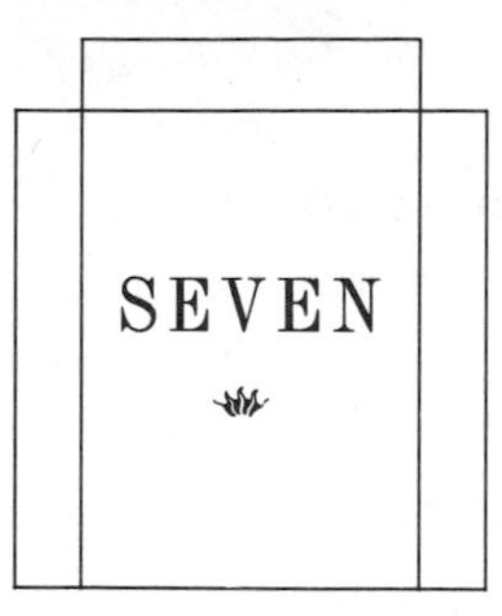


# *The Imaginative Lover*

I believe that underneath that strong exterior is a whole reservoir of romantic, sensual feelings waiting to be tapped. Release them and give yourself permission to experience the pleasure of being the one who turns your woman on. It doesn't have to be the rock 'n' roll star or movie heartthrob. You are the one she loves.

For all of you who would like to achieve more, or become more than you are at present, I have a wonderful, simple technique that will work instantaneously. It has worked for literally thousands of men just like you.

## PRETENDING HAS ITS REWARDS

The mind cannot distinguish between what is real and what is make-believe. Perception has nothing to do with reality. What we imagine can be as real to us as reality itself. Consequently, the way we act in real life can be determined beforehand by imagining a situation, then imagining the best possible action we could take. This principle is used extensively to train athletes, soldiers, and professional men.

In one behavioral study, basketball players were divided into three groups. One group was told to practice shooting baskets thirty minutes a day. The next was told to do nothing, and the third group was told to lie down for thirty minutes a day and picture themselves shooting perfect baskets. At the end of a month, the three groups were asked to shoot baskets, and the researchers found that the group that did nothing had fallen behind in their abilities, but the results of the other two groups were identical. The group that had spent time just imagining the perfect shot and the group that practiced daily had improved equally.

The military uses a variation of this technique to train their men. They simulate battle conditions and have their troops react accordingly, practicing until their reactions are almost automatic. Professional men are trained to deal with customers and clients, as well as with the people they will be supervising, well in advance of actual situations. The mind works as if these role-playing situations are real at the time, even though they aren't. Then, when faced with the actual experience, the mind is very comfortable thinking, "Oh, I remember this. It's nothing new. I've done this before."

Now let's use this same principle to become a better lover, a happier person, and a more secure human being.

When Kevin took my class, he was scared to death of women and especially of rejection. He had never dated in high school and was now in his senior year of college. He desperately wanted to ask a certain girl in one of his classes out for a date. But whenever he tried to approach her, his palms became sweaty, his heart began to beat faster, and his words choked in his throat. Disappointed and angry with himself, he would walk away from her feeling like a failure.

I asked Kevin to pretend for two weeks, thirty minutes each night before he fell asleep, that he was a "ladies' man." He was to think of himself as sexy, handsome, and successful, a man every woman in the school desired to date. In his fantasy, he was to have the phone ringing constantly, with women asking him out and he having to turn them down. He was to say to himself things like, "So many women to choose from, so little time," or "There's only so much of me to spread around. I have to be selective." Then he was to picture himself conversing with the woman of his dreams. He was charming, interesting, funny, and intriguing, and her response to him was extremely positive. He had to promise to carry this out every night for thirty minutes. He did, and the results were nothing less than miraculous. He spent a total of seven hours (fourteen days times thirty minutes) tricking his mind.

I received a call from him as soon as he put what had only existed in his mind into reality. He was so excited, he couldn't contain himself. Not only had he been able to talk to the woman in his class, but they had set a study date for one evening before their next exam.

Any man can become a romantic lover, no matter what his upbringing, fears, or lack of motivation. How? By pretending you already are the man of your woman's dreams. You are the perfect man who knows how to cater to a woman's every need.

- If you are coming home from work and the last thing you feel is loving, pretend you are. Give her a pretend passionate kiss hello.

- If you are a nervous, insecure person, pretend you have all the confidence and self-esteem that a person can possess and sweep her off her feet.
- If you have no imagination, pretend you are the most creative man on earth. By the way, every little boy has a terrific imagination. What child did not pretend to be a soldier, fireman, or doctor? (Remember wanting to play doctor and being told to stop it?) You are imaginative; you just haven't used that creativity for some time.
- If you lack motivation, ask yourself, "If I were motivated, what would I do?" and act accordingly.
- If you no longer love your mate, pretend you do. How would you act if you were having an affair with her? I know you can do it, and when you do, you will actually feel as if you're having an affair.

Use your imagination, see yourself doing these things, and you'll find that *your pretend self will become real.*

Homer decided to take a chance and become daring and adventurous. He told the class, "My wife is always the one who has planned surprises for me. I've always thought of myself as a very practical, analytical type of person, and we've both come to accept the fact that I'm just not imaginative. Well, this week I decided to try Ellen's theory. I imagined that I was a favorite actor of mine, Clark Gable. I thought about how he would treat a woman, and the rest became quite simple. I went to a department store and bought myself a silk robe, an ascot, and some new cologne. Then I went to a nearby Italian restaurant and ordered a complete takeout dinner for two. My wife almost fainted when she came home from work and saw the candlelight dinner and me all dressed up for her. She's still talking about that night to all her friends. The wonderful part of this role-playing was that I really did get excited, and for the first time, I really felt that I was capable of being romantic."

Perry and his wife pretended they were on their first date. "I actually started getting butterflies in my stomach as the night progressed. It was so refreshing, and our lovemaking was fantastic." We all laughed when he added that after he and his wife of nineteen years made love, he called her a slut for going to bed on their first date! That smart woman replied, "I couldn't help myself. You were so sexy that I had no control over my body. This is the first time I've ever done anything like this."

So become an actor and wind up the hero in your mate's life. What will start as a pretense will become real for you. I guarantee it.

## CONFIDENTIAL

**These next few pages are to be read only if you are a man who is ready for an exotic adventure and an evening you'll never forget.**

As you read this section, you might be tempted to say, "This is definitely not me. I just don't do things like this." If you find yourself feeling this way, remember my previous advice: *Don't be you, be someone else.* You are now going to pretend that you are a man who is exciting, sexy, artistic, witty, and desirable. I promise that your "pretend self" will have no trouble at all with this kind of wonderful experimentation. Don't let your "real self" ruin the adventure you are about to have.

## BE HER FANTASY

There's a saying, "We always want what we don't have." If you are a man who always wears a suit to work, change your image for one night. Be a soldier, an astronaut, a doctor, a fireman, or a policeman. You'd be surprised at how many women get turned on by uniforms. They can be rented for an evening very inexpensively at a costume shop. Imagine her shock if you secretly change into this costume when she least expects it. Here's your chance to be a football or baseball player as well. Costumes have a way of transforming people into the characters they're pretending to be. Certainly, Halloween is an example of a holiday where many men allow their creative, imaginative sides to come out. The most conservative men become the most outrageous characters one night a year. You don't need a holiday to give you permission to have fun and create a memory. You'll surprise yourself at what a clever man you are capable of becoming. Let your personality fit your outfit, and play the role the entire evening.

- If you are a pirate, look for the treasure of love together.
- If you are a police officer, arrest her and book her into your bedroom.
- If you are a fireman, rescue her from the flames of boredom and routine.
- If you are a soldier, protect her from the attack of monotony and predictability.

- If you are an astronaut, take her to the moon and back with you.
- If you are a doctor, examine her very carefully to find out what's wrong.

If you don't wear a business suit at work then buy a three-piece suit and play millionaire tycoon or just a business professional. Let her be your secretary, or better yet, your business partner, and have fun arranging a situation where you are so attracted to her that you can't seem to concentrate on your work.

Here's the secret of not having a boring relationship. *The best way to avoid a boring relationship is not to be a boring person.* Take responsibility for boredom and don't sit around waiting for her to provide the excitement. Some men keep changing partners because they are so easily bored; they're always looking for new women to entertain them. You can provide the excitement and unpredictability that is vital in a committed relationship.

Some of the braver men in my class who have tried these suggestions have reported wonderful results.

> Tony said he couldn't remember when he had a better time. He came home at noon, rang the front doorbell and pretended he was a TV repairman. He and his wife starred in their own "soaps" that day.
>
> Les said he and his wife laughed so hard, they probably added at least ten years to their lives. He was a frog in search of a princess. When kissed he would turn into a handsome prince and get rid of the evil spell that was cast on him many years ago.

Monty said he found a whole new dimension to his personality that he never knew existed when he and his wife acted out *Beauty and the Beast.*

Vince admitted that he and his wife made love in the backyard in an old tent because he was a soldier.

Kenneth revealed that he and his wife spent the night in his kid's teepee, since he chose to be an Indian.

I know, and now all these men know, too, that if a couple is laughing and having fun, their sex life improves one hundred percent. Once you get the hang of this, you'll be able to create a whole new range of experiences in a relationship that has become a little too familiar and predictable.

Stan wrote his wife a note telling her to go to a neighborhood bar; a secret admirer was waiting for her there. When she arrived, he spent the whole evening trying to pick her up. When she finally succumbed to his charms, he was the envy of men both to the left and right of him, even impressing the unsuspecting bartender! More important, he was surprised at how triumphant he felt as he left with his prize package—his own wife.

Phil, who had always envied the high school quarterback, finally got his chance with the most popular girl in school. He rented a football uniform for himself and a cheerleading costume, complete with pompons, for his wife. He said he had the best time living out a fantasy he had had for years. The unexpected surprise was that his wife got to be a cheerleader—her own teen-age dream come true!

Jeanie was full of embarrassment and delight when Lloyd

came strolling into her office dressed as a policeman. As it turned out, the whole office knew of his plans to surprise her and whisk her away for a weekend to celebrate their twentieth anniversary. He had made all the plans, which included a call to her boss requesting that Jeanie have Friday afternoon off. He made the most of his costume, arresting her on the spot and, of course, reading her her "rights."

He said, "You've been accused of spending too much time with the children and not enough with me. You have the right to remain silent. You also have the right to spend a romantic weekend with me. You have the right to a hotel room. If you do not have one, then a suite will be provided for you. Anything you say now will be used later to make love to you." Then out came a pair of toy handcuffs, and away they went.

Lloyd not only created a memory that will last forever, he also made Jeanie the envy of every woman in her office.

Jay was brave enough to rent a doctor's garb for himself and a nurse's uniform for his girlfriend. He left her uniform on the bed, and when she got home, there was a note waiting asking her to put on the outfit and meet him in front of a local hospital. They had fun playing the game he always wanted to play when he was a little boy!

Here's another secret few men know. *Inside every woman, no matter how strong and capable, there's a little girl waiting to come out and play.* Be playful with her and encourage her to participate, to become a little girl again, at least for a while. The man who is able to release that little girl through a sense of humor becomes indispensable in her life. Go for it. You both deserve it!

## LET YOUR MIND ESCAPE EVEN WHEN YOUR BODY CAN'T

"Men are not imaginative enough," says Eileen, a woman in her late thirties. "They always expect the woman to come up with new ideas, and frankly, I'm fed up. Just once, I'd like to see the man be creative."

Okay, here's another chance. You won't need a costume for this, only your imagination. Many times, a long-term relationship becomes boring and routine because your mate is so familiar and you get into the habit of making love in the same place at the same time, all the time. Sometimes the answer is not in changing mates or going to different locations, but just in pretending that you are somewhere else with your mate, and the two of you have just met. If your body can't escape routine and boredom, at least your mind can. Try some of these skits with her. You'll be absolutely amazed at the effect they can have on your everyday life.

## STAR IN YOUR OWN CREATED ROLE

Ask her to pretend along with you. You are the hero, and she's the heroine, and both of you are whoever you want to be. You can have action, glamour, excitement, sex, love, anything you want, and it takes nothing more than a little imagination. The memories with the one you love will always be there, along with a closeness that you will always cherish.

Here are some ideas for plots. Try more than just one of them, and remember, these are just descriptions of the scene. What you do with them from there is entirely up to you and her.

### Prisoner of Love

You are a prisoner, accused of a heinous crime. She is a young, sophisticated lawyer who has come to see you because she's the only person in the world who believes in your innocence. And, of course, you both fall madly in love.

### You're Under Seducement

You are a police officer who has just stopped a speeding car. You realize that she's trying to seduce you as you are writing the ticket. You try to ignore this lady's beautiful legs and captivating eyes as long as you can, but after all, you are only human.

### Vidal Sassoon

You are the owner of a salon, and she is sitting demurely in the chair waiting for her freshly washed hair to be blow dried. The conversation starts out innocently enough, but the more you dry, the more wildly attracted you are. What can you do to win your way into her heart?

### Teach Me Tonight

You are a professor. As you are giving your lecture, one of your students (guess who?) starts flirting with you. She's making all these extremely suggestive gestures, which makes it terribly hard for you to concentrate on your topic, so it really is imperative that you keep her after class.

### Keeping in Shape

You are both working out in a gym, and you can't keep your eyes off her. She is such a vision of beauty as she rides the excercycle and works the machines that it consumes all your strength just to watch her. You must tell her, you *must!*

### Play with Me

You are sitting at a play minding your own business when a strange woman sits down next to you. You can't help smelling her wonderful perfume and noticing a shapely knee, but the play really is good, and you really do want to see it through, but wait. What is this? What is this pressure you begin to feel against your leg . . . ?

### Date Me

You are both in the lobby of a video dating service waiting to be taped. You find each other most attractive, and in the next ten minutes there is a good chance that you are both going to tear up your applications.

### Give Me a Loan

You are a loan officer, and she's a successful woman who needs $1 million to expand her business. You have to ask her many, many questions to determine whether you can give her the money. She's willing to do anything to get that loan.

### Doctor, Doctor

She's a young, beautiful doctor, and you need a physical exam in the worst way. It seems you've been having trouble lately with all sorts of things, and you really need somebody to take a look at you, somebody who cares, somebody who can fix all your problems.

### Home, Sweet Home

You're strangers, and you both want the same apartment. It's perfect, and you both want to take it immediately. Is it possible that you could compromise?

### Dancing in the Dark

It is 1935, and you are young and inexperienced. The lights are low, and the Gramophone is playing a slow tune. Even though you are nervous and shy, you ask her to dance. As she comes into your arms, you can tell that she is as excited as you are. Before you know it, you are Fred Astaire and she is Ginger Rogers.

### At Your Service

You are young and naïve, delivering pizza for a living. She answers the door, and look out!

### A Winning Hand

You are in a casino in Las Vegas. Both of you are at the blackjack table winning a great deal of money. You strike up a conversation, and soon find that you are bringing each other luck. How much more luck will you have?

### After the Storm

This one is wonderful to use just after you've had an argument. You are very much in love with each other, but, unfortunately, you are both married to other people, and you are having a desperate affair. Here's your chance to complain about that awful wife, and she can complain about her terrible husband. You both count your blessings that for at least a few short times a week, you can escape and be together.

## MOVING INTO THE BEDROOM

Everything I've talked about so far has been taking place outside the bedroom. If you have been sincerely trying to be a more daring, exciting, sensuous, imaginative mate, I'm going to assume you now have a woman who is much more receptive to making love with you.

Now, this is an area where your mate really needs your help. Chances are, she is not as comfortable with her own sexuality as you are. It is only through your tenderness, warmth, acceptance, and knowledge that you can become her greatest teacher. You can help release her femininity, help her become a more creative lover, and ultimately allow her to experience sexual fulfillment. It is through her responsiveness to you that you will experience the ultimate pleasure.

It is not easy for some women to let go of their inhibitions, and a great deal of patience and affection is necessary on your part. Encourage her to appreciate her body as you do. If she's embarrassed to get undressed in front of you, don't insist. Let her get under the covers and, with your words, reinforce over and over how much you love her body. Above all, say something to her, something of endearment, of assurance, of caring, and of the love you have for her. Then tell her she's sexy, that she turns you on. You may have to begin in the dark, but little by little, as she gains more confidence, you can add candlelight or red light bulbs to create a romantic atmosphere.

I once heard someone say that a man can be compared to a pile of dry leaves, while a woman is like charcoal. Strike a match to the leaves, and they catch fire immediately. The charcoal takes much longer, but eventually both the leaves and the charcoal will be equally hot.

As a man, there's a good probability that you can experience sexual arousal and climax with relative ease. This is not the case for many women. It takes much longer. Many women have said that it takes at least thirty to sixty minutes before they are ready. You may be thinking, "That's an eternity. I'll never be able to last that long." Erase that thought from your head and replace it with, "Wow, that's exciting. I'll have one hour to arouse, excite, and stimulate her." The ultimate challenge for you is to postpone your own pleasure in return for a much greater sense of satisfaction when you both experience sexual fulfillment at the end of lovemaking.

It's important to add here that sometimes having a "quickie" is appropriate and exciting. The spontaneity that occurs if you should suddenly have an urge while driving in the car, taking a walk in the woods, at the beach, or even on a football field late at night can be absolutely wonderful. Many times, arousal is heightened for both partners when the element of surprise is added. It's also important to understand that there is quite a difference between having sex and making love. They are two very different things, and you must know how to do both.

So let's get back to the art of making love to a woman.

Usually a woman loves to be massaged. It's important for her to relax. Massage her back, neck, feet, and hands, and by all means, this is the time to tell her how pretty she is, how much you love her, and what a difference she makes in your life. (Of course, this is not the only time you tell her these things.) Brushing her hair also contributes to relaxing her.

When you start your lovemaking, it is important that you don't begin by stroking her intimate parts. You want to prepare her for this enjoyment later. Kissing, hugging, and cuddling are essential for her to become aroused. Stroking and being stroked is an exciting activity you both can enjoy. Don't cheat yourself out of the warmth and stimulation that touching each other produces.

When she becomes sufficiently aroused, after about thirty to sixty minutes of foreplay, then she's ready for more intimate caressing. The gentle stroking of her clitoris, along with kissing and stroking her breasts, will bring her to heightened sexual arousal that will then lead toward her having an orgasm.

Many men, and many women as well, are not aware that this part of the female body, the clitoris, corresponds to the male penis. It is one of the most sensitive parts of her body and must be stroked with care, but nonetheless needs to be stroked. Contrary to what some people think, she cannot have an orgasm by just inserting your penis into her vagina. There are very few nerve endings in her vagina. Years ago, experts believed that there were two types of orgasms, vaginal and clitoral. Today, we know that it is only through stimulating the clitoris that orgasm is possible.

## WHERE IT'S AT

The clitoris is relatively small and will feel like a little bump just above the entrance to her vagina. This tiny organ is located where the folds of the inner lips of the vulva come together. It is not inside her body. It is outside. If you are still not sure where it is, it might be fun to go together to your local library or purchase a book that has a detailed picture of a woman's body.

It's also important to note the following:

- If the stroking is too aggressive, too strong, or too rough, a woman's body will shut down.
- Since sex is in her head and not in bed for many women, if she's not receptive to lovemaking because there hasn't been sufficient arousal (or romance), her body will not respond.
- The size of a man's penis has little to do with giving a woman sexual fulfillment.
- It is not necessary or important for you to have an orgasm together. What is important is for each of you to enjoy the other and attend to each other's needs.
- For some women, having an orgasm is not that important. They prefer the closeness of the sexual union. They derive more satisfaction from holding, caressing, and kissing than the actual act of sex. Even if they do have an orgasm, they feel cheated if sufficient time hasn't been spent on feeling close to you.

There's irony in the fact that many men who are aggressive and just plain tough will have to abandon these traits and become tender, gentle, and kind if they want their mates to be responsive sexually. While, in general, there is a time and place for everything, if you want rough and tumble, go play football. She is different from you, both emotionally and physically.

Did you know that as a man, your body releases a chemical that causes you to feel sleepy after you make love? And while you're feeling sleepy, the wonderful woman lying beside you releases a hormone that makes her wide awake. She's basking in the afterglow and wants more cuddling, hugging, kisses, and intimate conversation, and you usually want nothing more than to close your eyes and drift off. But this sleepy feeling only lasts a few seconds, and if you could force yourself to stay awake, she'll feel like the luckiest woman alive to have a lover who hasn't left her.

Another physiological difference between the two of you is that the hormone levels in most men are highest in the morning. This is one of the reasons men generally wake up with an erection. For many women, however, arousal is easiest in the evening, because it's then that their hormone levels tend to be highest. If you are both aware of this difference, you can take turns pleasing each other. It is yet another way to show that you care.

Before you can touch the deepest core of a woman's sensuality and get to these playful and exciting evenings of wild abandon, it is important that you remember what you've learned from the previous chapters and put these things into practice daily. Tenderness, understanding, appreciation, and sensitivity can bring your relationship to a level that most people, both men and women, can only wish for. Show her that you have these traits in abundance, give them to her constantly, and you will make it difficult for your woman to keep her hands off you.

## ACTION ASSIGNMENT #7

1. Make the most of your pretend self. When you get home, give her a pretend passionate kiss hello and sweep her off her feet.
2. Give her advance notice of a future date that will be a very special evening for her.
3. Be daring and innovative. Let your imagination run wild. Be her fantasy and transform yourself into someone else for one evening.
4. Ask her to go shopping with you, then ask her to pick out some sexy underwear that she'd like to see you in.
5. Become the tender, sensitive lover she needs. One night this week, treat your lovemaking as an event in itself, not a prelude to sleep. Be gentle and take the time to make her happy and satisfied, then look for the glow in her cheeks the next morning.

Dear Ellen,

Thank you, thank you, thank you. As you know, Wallace and I are retired. We are both in our late sixties. Remember when we first agreed to take "Light Her Fire," and I called to tell you that my biggest concern was that he would be no fun to grow old with? Well, I want you to know that your class has exceeded all my expectations. The little acts of kindness that he now does every day have given me a whole new lease on life. I go to bed every night knowing I'm the luckiest woman alive to have this fantastic man next to me.

Love,
Mattie

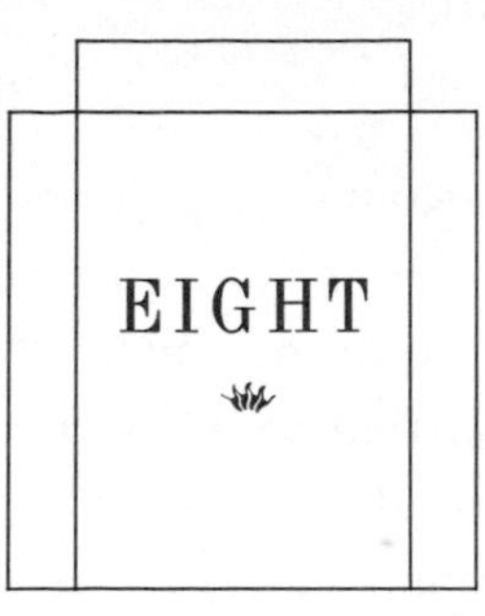

# EIGHT

# *Love Is*

I hear the most wonderful stories about what men have done to bring more happiness into their mates' lives. They are stories of uncommon kindness, craziness, self-sacrifice, and unbounded love, and in them are lessons that we all need to be constantly aware of. You not only have to say you love her, you need to show it, too, every chance you get.

I remember June telling everyone, with tears in her eyes, "When my back went out, I was rushed to the emergency room. After a week in traction, I was finally released. The doctor told me that I had to remain in bed for at least another week. I couldn't believe my eyes when I finally got comfortable under the covers. There was a brand-new TV with a remote control for me. My husband had spent half his paycheck so that I would be comfortable."

Virginia told us that she works for a telemarketing firm at night in her home. One day when she sat down, there was a telephone headset like the kind operators use that her husband had purchased without her knowing. He was concerned about how uncomfortable it was to hold a telephone receiver to her ear for many hours and how that would eventually put a strain on her neck.

Kerry, who is married to a construction worker, said, "On our anniversary, Marion gave me the shock of my life. He made all the arrangements to have us take our marriage vows again in the same church where we were married twenty-six years before. He bought a new suit, made our daughter the bridesmaid, and bought a huge corsage for me. When the ceremony was completed, we all went out to dinner, where I proceeded to cry tears of happiness all night long."

Lili said that one particular year, money had been a big problem in their marriage. She didn't get the promotion she was hoping for, and Dick had had some health problems that had caused him to miss work. To her amazement, her husband announced that they were going on a weekend vacation the following week. She, of course, asked him if he was crazy, because they had no money. He told her not to worry, that it was all taken care of. The following Saturday when all the bags were packed, he told her to close her eyes as he led her to the front door. When she opened it, there was a red carpet (he used a long roll of paper that was painted red) leading up to their camper. She thought immediately that this was going to be work, not a vacation. She discovered she was wrong. He had shopped for all the supplies, cleaned the entire camper, and packed it. When they got to their destination, he brought out a small table, a red-and-white checkered tablecloth, champagne, candles, and flowers. He cooked breakfast, lunch, and dinner for two days and did all the cleanup. He waited on her hand and foot. Lili told us it was the best time she had ever had.

Carolyn said she'd never forget New Year's Eve, 1989. At three that afternoon a white limousine pulled up in front of her house. "My husband handed me a large manila envelope and instructed my girlfriend and me to get into the limousine. Inside the envelope, we found pictures and a cassette tape. On the tape was the theme from *Mission Impossible,* with instructions to find our husbands. Our first stop was at a well-known department store in our area. You can't imagine our surprise when we were escorted to a dressing room filled with party dresses. My friend's size was on the left, and mine was on the right. We were told to pick out a dress, shoes, and accessories, then dress from head to toe in an hour and a half. Then we were taken by the limo to a hotel suite filled with two dozen roses, champagne, decorations, and music. To this day, I'm treated like a celebrity at that department store."

These wonderful, romantic men certainly know how to Light Her Fire!

I couldn't end this book, however, without sharing some of the little things that men do that mean so much to the women that love them. I know I've said it in past chapters, but I'll say it again. *Little things mean a lot.* Sure, it's wonderful to plan a great big display of your love, but it's very important to know that the small acts of tenderness and kindness daily also show a woman how much you love, respect, and appreciate her.

So here's a list composed by women who are motivated to Light His Fire, because they have men who know how to Light Her Fire.

LOVE IS . . . putting on the electric blanket before she gets into bed so that it's toasty warm for her.

LOVE IS . . . getting into the car a few minutes before her and saying, "I'll warm up the car for you, honey."

LOVE IS . . . putting your arm around her and asking if she's warm enough.

LOVE IS . . . calling her from work and asking if she needs anything from the grocery store on your way home.

LOVE IS . . . locking all the doors and windows at night to make sure she feels safe.

LOVE IS . . . bringing her a cup of coffee in the morning and putting it on her night table next to the bed.

LOVE IS . . . being extra quiet in the morning if you have to get up earlier than she does.

LOVE IS . . . not rustling papers in bed if you have a lot of reading to do when she's trying to sleep.

LOVE IS . . . calling her from work for no other reason than to tell her how much you love her.

LOVE IS . . . greeting her at the car to help her carry in the grocery bags.

LOVE IS . . . telling your friends in front of her how wonderful she is.

LOVE IS . . . leaving the house and garage lights on if she's coming home late.

LOVE IS . . . you getting out of bed to see why the dog is barking.

LOVE IS . . . asking her what program she'd like to see on TV.

LOVE IS . . . noticing how pretty she looks without her having to ask.

LOVE IS . . . helping her with the household chores such as vacuuming, dusting, cleaning, and doing the windows.

LOVE IS . . . helping her give the kids a bath and putting them to bed so she can relax.

LOVE IS . . . helping her take off her boots or zipping up her dress.

LOVE IS . . . helping her close the clasp of a necklace she wants to wear.

LOVE IS . . . shaving and showering before you make love to her.

LOVE IS . . . massaging her feet, back, neck, or hands after a long day.

LOVE IS . . . washing the dishes and cleaning up the kitchen after eating and letting her rest if she has prepared the meal.

LOVE IS . . . going with her to a doctor or dentist appointment if she's nervous.

LOVE IS . . . you picking her up at the hospital the day she's being discharged.

LOVE IS . . . remembering to put the toilet seat cover down when you're finished.

LOVE IS . . . cleaning out the hairs in the sink after you've shaved.

LOVE IS . . . being interested in knowing how her day was spent.

LOVE IS . . . getting up to feed the baby at 3:00 A.M.

LOVE IS . . . taking a long walk holding hands.

LOVE IS . . . getting her a refill for her drink at a social function.

LOVE IS . . . keeping a picture of her on your desk and in your wallet.

LOVE IS . . . writing her a poem or letter telling her how proud you are to be with her and why.

LOVE IS . . . never taking your eyes off her to stare at another woman, no matter how attractive.

LOVE IS . . . apologizing if you are wrong and saying nothing if you are right.

LOVE IS . . . flirting with her when you're at a party.

LOVE IS . . . taking her phone calls when she's tired and telling them she'll call back.

LOVE IS . . . every once in a while filling her car with gas and having it washed.

LOVE IS . . . sometimes acting cheerful and pleasant even when you don't feel that way.

LOVE IS . . . turning off the alarm every morning and turning to her with, "I love you."

LOVE IS . . . putting on a bow tie and draping a large napkin over your arm and becoming a waiter who serves the dinner. If she tries to get up for something, say, "No, no, madam, I will get it!"

LOVE IS . . . scheduling her in your appointment book for a nice long lunch.

LOVE IS . . . cuddling together as you reminisce about the good times you've had together.

LOVE IS . . . asking her to marry you again on the day of your anniversary.

LOVE IS . . . saying, "Come here and sit on my lap," having her put her arms around your neck, and starting to kiss like teen-agers again.

LOVE IS . . . asking her to dance right there in your living room, kitchen, or den.

LOVE IS . . . spending at least one night alone together.

LOVE IS . . . sharing a dream together—picking out a vacation you'd like to take or the house you want—and talking about it together. Cut out pictures and start an album of "future dreams."

LOVE IS . . . sharing a lazy day together, renting some movies, taking a nap, reading, and just resolving to be together "doing nothing" all day.

LOVE IS . . . taking a shower or bath together.

LOVE IS . . . being there to greet her at the airport when her flight comes in and helping carry her bags.

LOVE IS . . . helping her map out directions to an appointment and even making a trial run the day before if necessary.

LOVE IS . . . renting a romantic movie you know she would like.

These simple acts of kindness make a woman feel loved, cared for, appreciated, and special. Begin today. Take one idea and try it out. See how easy it really is to ignite the flames of passion and excitement in the woman you love.

# CONCLUSION

We've come to the end of the book, but I hope it's just the beginning for you.

You deserve to have a woman who loves you with all her heart. By now, you've learned that it won't happen by chance or luck or by being in the right place at the right time. It will happen through your growing awareness that her needs and requirements may be different from yours. When you give her the kind of strength, understanding, tenderness, and sensitivity she needs, you'll get her respect, admiration, support, and passion in return.

There is so much in life over which you have no control. Your love life is not one of these areas. You can have complete control there, but you must decide that you want to have all that a woman is capable of giving you.

Living with and loving a woman can be the most challenging and rewarding experience you'll ever have. The deep sense of satisfaction that comes when a woman is at your side has no equal. She's there to give you a sense of worth, to share in your successes and failures, and to confirm your manhood.

Join the thousands of men who are now thought of as lucky when others see their relationships. They've learned that luck is hard work that has finally paid off.

I want you to have the ultimate payoff, a woman who worships the ground you walk on and who would do anything to make you happy. Prove to her that the man of her dreams, her Prince Charming, her knight in shining armor, her hero, has finally come true because of you.

I wish you all the love, happiness, and fulfillment that you deserve.

Love,
Ellen

P.S. I'd love to hear about some of the fabulous changes that I'm sure have occurred in your life after you've read this book. Please write to:

LHF Enterprises
P.O. Box 1511
El Toro, CA 92630

# ABOUT THE AUTHOR

ELLEN KREIDMAN is the founder of the courses "Light His Fire" and "Light Her Fire." For the past nine years she has been a dynamic public speaker who has motivated and educated thousands of men and women. She has a combined B.A. in psychology and education. She has had a twenty-four-year-long love affair with her husband and has three children. Ms. Kreidman lives in El Toro, California.